YOGA
— FOR —
MENOPAUSE
— AND —
BEYOND

YOGA FOR MENOPAUSE AND BEYOND

GUIDING TEACHERS AND STUDENTS THROUGH CHANGE

NIAMH DALY

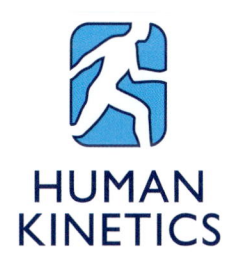

HUMAN KINETICS

Copyright © 2025 by Niamh Daly. All rights reserved. No portion of this book, except for brief review, may be reproduced, stored in a retrieval system, or transmitted in any form or by any means—electronic, mechanical, photocopying, recording, or otherwise—without the written permission of the publisher. For information, contact Human Kinetics.

First published in 2025 by
Human Kinetics
1607 N. Market Street, Champaign, Illinois 61820

United States and International
Website: **US.HumanKinetics.com**
Email: info@hkusa.com
Phone: 1-800-747-4457

Canada
Website: **Canada.HumanKinetics.com**
Email: info@hkcanada.com

Illustrations Niamh Daly
Photographs Sharon Smith
Editor Simon Coury
Text Design Medlar Publishing Solutions Pvt Ltd., India
Cover Design Chris Fulcher
Printed and Bound in the United States of America

Medical Disclaimer
This publication is written and published to provide accurate and authoritative information relevant to the subject matter presented. It is published and sold with the understanding that the author and publishers are not engaged in rendering legal, medical, or other professional services by reason of their authorship or publication of this work. If medical or other expert assistance is required, the services of a competent professional person should be sought.

British Library Cataloging-in-Publication Data
A CIP record for this book is available from the British Library

Library of Congress Cataloging-in-Publication Data
Names: Daly, Niamh, author.
Title: Yoga for menopause and beyond : guiding teachers and students
  through change / Niamh Daly.
Description: Champaign, Illinois : Human Kinetics, 2025. | Includes
  bibliographical references and index.
Identifiers: LCCN 2024007115 (print) | LCCN 2024007116 (ebook) | ISBN
  9781718236912 (paperback) | ISBN 9781718236943 (epub) | ISBN
  9781718236950 (pdf)
Subjects: LCSH: Menopause--Popular works. | Hatha yoga--Therapeutic use. |
  Middle-aged women--Health and hygiene. | BISAC: HEALTH & FITNESS / Yoga
  | HEALTH & FITNESS / Exercise / Stretching
Classification: LCC RG186 .D27 2025 (print) | LCC RG186 (ebook) | DDC
  615.8/24--dc23/eng/20240324
LC record available at https://lccn.loc.gov/2024007115
LC ebook record available at https://lccn.loc.gov/2024007116

ISBN: 978-1-7182-3691-2
10 9 8 7 6 5 4 3 2 1
E9855

*To my mother Aoibheann (1933–1985), wishing
I'd known you in my adulthood, to express
my understanding and respect for you, my interest
in your life experiences. I wonder if we would have
spoken together of the joy and pain of womanhood,
and held each other in the complex beauty of mothering.*

*Remembering also my father Robert (1928–1986),
who showed his beloved all those qualities,
and held her in it all.*

*To my daughters Evie and Ríona, the centres of my heart.
I hope that the work I am doing now will contribute
to a fear-free, empowered journey through the stages
of their lives.*

CONTENTS

ACKNOWLEDGMENTS	9
INTRODUCTION	13
A note about inclusion	15

CHAPTER 1
THE BIOCHEMISTRY OF MENOPAUSE — 17

The main players	18
Estrogen	18
Progesterone	19
Follicle-stimulating hormone	19
The supporting roles	20
The stages of menopause	20
The late reproductive stage (LRS) and perimenopause	20
Postmenopause	24
The health implications of menopause	25
Thyroid health	26
Lung function	26
The role of stress	27

CHAPTER 2
RESEARCH INTO YOGA FOR MENOPAUSE — 31

The evidence for yoga	31
Is this evidence enough?	36
Selling yoga for menopause	38
A new approach to yoga for menopause?	39

CHAPTER 3
A CLASS, REIMAGINED — 43

a) **An opening circle, enriched**	43
The late reproductive stage and early perimenopause	43
Perimenopause	44
Postmenopause	45
b) **A constant: language reconsidered**	46
Your teaching language	48
A trauma perspective on language and teaching	50
c) **A warm-up, hard-wired for pleasure**	55
Somatic movement	55
Pleasure and the feel-good hormones	63
d) **Asana, responsive to change**	70
Exercise in general	72
Functional yoga in the stages of menopause	73
Stretching	74
e) **Rest times, revalued**	89
Some favourite restoratives	93
Yoga Nidra	96
Shavasana	97
f) **Meditation and breath, renewed**	99
Seated positions	99
Pranayama	100
Guided meditations	102
Perspective shifts	106
Cognitive behavioral therapy	107

CHAPTER 4
ENHANCING YOGA FOR MENOPAUSE HEALTH — 109

a) **Bones** — 109
- The changing biology — 109
- Can yoga help? — 111
- How yoga can help — 111
- Protection first — 112
- Yoga for bone health — 118
- Stimulating bone — 118
- Posture and balance — 127
- Support outside yoga—nutrition — 127

b) **Brain** — 128
- The changing biology — 128
- How yoga can help — 129
- The vagus nerve — 130
- Stimulating the brain — 132
- Support outside yoga — 135

c) **Pelvic floor** — 142
- The changing biology — 142
- How yoga can help — 143
  - *Mula bandha* — 144
  - *Uddiyana bandha or hypopressives* — 145
- Staying connected — 151
- Support outside yoga — 153

CHAPTER 5
A JOURNEY, SUPPORTED — 155

a) **Perimenopause, symptoms addressed** — 155
- Sleep, hot flashes, and anxiety — 156
- Changing mood — 163
- Energy and focus — 168
- Aching joints — 171
- Weight gain — 172
- Libido changes — 174

b) **Protecting health** — 177
- Digestive health — 177
- The liver — 181
- Heart health — 183
- Systemic inflammation — 185
- The lymphatic system — 186
- Blood sugar regulation — 188

CHAPTER 6
FOOD AND MEDICINE — 191

Nutrition — 191
- Diet and dieting — 191
- Emotional eating — 192
- Phytoestrogens — 192
- Nutrition for menopause condensed — 193

Menopause hormone therapy — 194

Your responsibilities — 197

AFTERWORD — 199

In summary — 199
- What would a yoga for menopause class look like? — 200

My hopes — 201
- For yoga and its teachers — 201
- For women and for my daughters — 202

REFERENCES — 205

INDEX — 217

PEER REVIEWS — 223

ACKNOWLEDGMENTS

With thanks to my daughters, Evie and Ríona, who may or may not have noticed my explorer's journey through perimenopause and how it impassioned, inspired, and impatiented me! I had reason to apologize to them many times, while also trying to make my needs clear, and to make space for me. Then, while I was writing this book, they put up with my "Hmm? What? Em … sorry, did you say something?" and some burnt dinners, as I typed and parented all at once! Thanks to their dad, Simon, who put up with all of the above too!

Thank you to Helena Walsh who, mid-conversation, transformed me from feeling this task was too big and my voice too insignificant, to knowing I had to—and could—bring to the yoga world my passionate convictions about this deeply important topic. I started bringing this book together moments later with fire in my belly and unstoppable stamina. Friend and mentor, without the "Yes! Now!" she ignited in me that day, this book might have remained in my head and the training manual of my Yoga teacher training (YTT), and never been transformed into this much richer and, I hope, long-term support for teachers and their students.

To Petra Fulham, deep gratitude. Through our friendship and work-partnership she has been instrumental in countless ways including enriching my knowledge, enlightening me as to how research can be analyzed, trusted, and/or critiqued, and helping me more keenly see how what I say can impact people in ways I had never considered.

To my editor, Simon Coury: "No, really?!" And "Wow, thank you!" I am an organic teacher, evident in the first draft which was passionate with lots of great content, but entirely unstructured. He put manners on this book. I was sometimes devastated and wondered should I have instead employed a half-baked editor! But he would (after looking at me with bewilderment as to my lack of structural skill) hear what I needed and help me feel capable of addressing what should be done. If this book is easy to make sense of, repeats itself only when necessary and has a structure that facilitates you to learn in reasonable increments, it is his fault!

Thank you to my peers in the menopause and/or yoga worlds who reviewed full drafts and/or sections of this book:

To consultant endocrinologist and author Dr Annice Mukherjee for her review of the section on hormone therapy and on the biochemistry of menopause. It has been a stabilizing relief to know her. I reached out to her in desolation about the medicalization and fear-inducing narrative of menopause that exploded after the airing of a documentary in 2021. She gave her valued time and contributed to my YTT, patiently responding to all my questions since! Her mentorship is the reason I feel able to stand with conviction behind what I say about MHT/HRT in this book, in the YTT and with clients. Without her I may have given up trying to help women with my no-false-promises approach in the face of the polarization and scaremongering we have seen in the media in the early 2020s.

To Tiffany Cruikshank, a skilled, outside-the-box trainer of teachers, who received an early, messy draft, patiently stopping mid-read and started again when I was ready to give her what you are reading here today. I must have seemed like such a flake! I am immensely grateful that she never seemed in the least bit miffed.

To Mary Flaherty, who was also the recipient of multiple drafts and didn't bat an eye. I am indebted to her for her peer review, but also for her years of research and the book she created that I only stumbled upon a few months ago. It is an incredible resource, and her keen eye was one I was so glad to have on my book.

Thanks also to my colleague-turned-friend Dr Jennifer Huber RD for her review of the nutrition and symptoms section. She was encouraging and also a grounding force, reminding me of how quickly research moves on.

Thanks to Rebekah Rotstein, who reviewed and offered tweaks to the section on bones. She is an excellent educator who really knows her stuff. Exacting but respectful, serious but open, and generous with her time and suggestions.

Thanks to the immensely knowledgeable Kim Vopni, who reviewed the section on pelvic floor health ("This is really great!" she said) and contributed to my YTT. As The Vagina Coach, she is empowering women by taking vaginas and pelvic floors out of the shadows.

A huge thanks to the intuitive, creative and intelligent yoga teacher Aoife Ní Mhurchú, who read that early, messy draft, essentially with a new-born at her breast, and gave me feedback that was at once reassuring and also astute and enlightening. She has made this book an easier read for you.

Thank you to my dear, generous sister Áine who modeled for the application of touch photos. She was the very first person who, on a mountain at sunrise, led me through a sun-salutation. Without her, there may have been no yoga for me!

Thank you to the articulate and supportive Fiona Daly, sister, psychotherapist, and sex and relationship counselor, who contributed her wisdom and expertise to the section on libido changes.

ACKNOWLEDGMENTS

To Sundar Maruthu, who took my word document and turned it into what you see here. I had no idea it was possible for it to be so beautiful to behold and to hold.

To Jon Hutchings, thank you for being reachable and for taking my first email seriously. I had become dismayed in my search for a publisher who would allow me the opportunity to articulate the need for this book person-to-person. He saw the need, and nurtured patiently this project (and my total lack of knowledge about publishing procedure!). More, he honoured it, spending untold hours ensuring it was as good as it could be. Even when I thought it couldn't be improved, he improved it!

Thank you to everyone at Human Kinetics. I am deeply honoured that a company with such integrity have taken on this book. It is niche (more than it should be!), so I know it's a decision that won't have been easy. Thanks to Jason who liaised with Jon and me, especially for his patience and help with finalizing the subtitle and the cover, and for bringing my various ideas to his colleagues so that these decisions were made with a background of great expertise.

To all my siblings, in gratitude for your presence and love. We have carried each other always. But more: I leaned, and you carried me, supporting my mental health during my perimenopause, in ways that have been both obvious and unaccountable to us all.

And thank you to some my teachers over the years, who may have no idea how much they have influenced me. Especially Marlene ffrench Mullen, Donna Farhi, Lisa Petersen, Gil Hedley, Sarah Lo, and John Sharkey.

INTRODUCTION

A woman's life in perimenopause and postmenopause is worth living, and worth living well. As difficult as it can be, perimenopause could be seen as a gift. It shows a woman what needs to be done. Along with the biochemical facts of hormonal changes, it is a time when the urgings of her body become louder and louder until she can no longer ignore them.

When she listens to what is actually being pleaded for by her exceptional, but undeniably human body, she gets the opportunity to respond in ways that make her present more comfortable, and her future more strong, reliable, alive, energized, and confident.

If she ignores the new environment of her organism, she may struggle more, lose opportunities for self-care, and live a life in judgement of her changing capabilities and in regret for the passage of time.

If we as yoga teachers ignore the effects of natural hormonal changes and how the way a woman cares for herself on every level often needs to change, we may unwittingly encourage our student to ignore her needs too. Offering yoga that is tailored to menopause and the years beyond signals to our students that their changing needs matter, can be addressed, and be skillfully and effectively supported.

This book is a menu of practices and strategies for teachers, female or male, all based on researched elements brought together into *Yoga for Menopause and Beyond*.

This book will help you to understand exactly how menopause affects women (physically, biochemically, mentally, emotionally, and socially), to see how some elements of yoga are tailor-made for supporting the female body in these stages, to see how some elements might be detrimental, and to see also how yoga may benefit from some sympathetic additions.

On the menu:

- Know, as a yoga teacher, that what you are teaching is, from a research-based perspective, truly supporting your students as they are now, not how they used to be.
- Enhance your understanding of what the body, brain, and spirit are experiencing through the different stages.

- Hear more accurately what it is that the body needs.
- Develop your ability to respond to women's symptoms in ways that ease rather than intensify them.
- Learn how to protect your student's health while her body is in a tricky process of change.
- Perfect small shifts to enhance her day-to-day and future wellbeing.
- Empower yourself and your students with perspectives on change, age, and self-value.
- Change the way you see women and their place in the world through the years.
- Help women feel free and empowered to take up the space they deserve.

As a yoga teacher since 2004, a nutrition and health coach and a Pilates instructor, I have, since 2015, been making the stages of menopause my specialist subject. Because women were expressing that they felt neglected, inaccurately supported, and unheard by all their providers of health and wellness support, the huge gap in education for yoga teachers about menopause troubled me.

All women who reach their 40s, or 50s at the oldest, *will* experience menopause, whereas only a proportion of women will ever birth a baby, and most will spend as much or more time in perimenopause and in postmenopause than pregnant and post-partum combined.

There are multiple important trainings educating yoga teachers about the needs of pregnancy and how to help support pregnant women, modules on which are often included even in entry-level teacher trainings. There are trainings in teaching yoga to teens, to children, and to the chair-bound. Niche areas!

So, I began to change this unacceptable state of affairs by developing my Certificate in Teaching Yoga for the Stages of Menopause and launching it in 2020. In subsequent years I developed menopause awareness courses for fitness and wellness professionals, and for psychotherapists and counsellors.

Since 2021, there has been a surge of wider interest in the struggles of perimenopause, support for the postmenopausal woman, and the education of medical and wellness professionals to offer this support appropriately. The world is waking up!

I call my graduating teachers, the women who worked so hard in the 2010s and 2020s to put menopause on the medical, social, workplace, wellness, fitness, and mental-healthcare maps, and myself, the Menopause Mavericks! A determined number of advocates, and I in my little yoga patch, have, in small or seismic ways, helped to create a generation more informed and empowered to take their midlife wellbeing into their own hands, demanding clarity and relevant support for their changing bodies.

I believe the yoga world needs to come up to speed with the medical and wellness worlds! By taking up this book, you are part of a new movement that will see the needs of menopause considered and embraced by yoga as it continues to develop.

I thank you for choosing me to be one of your resources to support the women in your classes.

A NOTE ABOUT INCLUSION

All the information in this book is relevant to those whose reduction of estrogen and progesterone has occurred or is beginning to occur, including young women experiencing early menopause, or women of any age whose medical treatments and/or surgeries have hastened the onset of perimenopause. Though in these situations there will need to be more cautious medical intervention, this book can still support them.

Further, I will mostly use the term "women," even though I am aware that there is an experience of menopause symptoms in people who have transitioned or are transitioning from female to male, and that people who have had/have ovaries, and who identify as male, will also experience the difficulties of perimenopause.

However, I have educated myself in, and primarily address, the biochemistry and social implications of peri/menopause from the perspective of average-onset female reproductive aging. I also address early menopause and menopause induced by surgical or medical treatment. The biochemistry is similar in all these cases, but the speed of hormonal change, severity of symptoms, level of health risks, and external contributing factors differ.

I would like to acknowledge that I do not yet feel skilled enough to educate teachers or individuals in a skillful way about the biopsychosocial impacts of treatment to transition from female to male, or the consequences when a male-to-female transgender person reaches a time when their hormone interventions need to be changed. Therefore I use the terms "woman" and "female" throughout this book.

The experiences of the neuro-diverse are also in my mind, and there are people researching the differences and similarities of the menopause as experienced by those who are not neuro-typical from a psychosocial aspect. To date, I am aware that for the neuro-diverse menopause can be more difficult than for the neuro-typical. Again, many of the practices in this book are still of potential value.

For people with mobility issues, the practices are mostly usable and/or adaptable by a skilled and creative teacher.

Lastly, I am aware of considerably different experiences of menopause, and differing health risks, depending on race and culture. Again, the practices in this book seek to support the universality of the biochemical changes of the reduction of estrogen and progesterone. However some of the writing regarding life-experiences may not be relevant to people in some cultures, of some ethnicities, and/or those with added difficulties of disability, neurodiversity, and/or gender diversity.

I hereby acknowledge my limitations.

Sanskrit
I mostly use English names commonly associated with asana. This is because some physical practices in the book are from different movement modalities and do not have Sanskrit names, and because I add elements to some postures that are not directly from yoga but are of my own invention. I use mostly Sanskrit (and some English) names of other yogic practices.

CHAPTER 1
THE BIOCHEMISTRY OF MENOPAUSE

Menopause is a word used to cover many phases that can occur over decades. However, menopause is essentially one day! Diagnosable only in retrospect, it's the day when your periods cease permanently, determined after one year without menstrual bleeding. The average age at which this happens is currently 51. The World Health Organization describes menopause as 'the end of monthly menstruation (also known as a menstrual period or "period") due to loss of ovarian follicular function' (WHO, 2022).

Leading up to menopause, the levels of a woman's reproductive hormones begin to change. There is a stage known as the late reproductive stage (LRS) that is characterized by barely noticeable variations in the menstrual cycle, and some symptoms. Next comes perimenopause, sometimes known as the menopause transition (MT), which is a time of variable menstrual length and a high number of possible symptoms. Menopause leads directly into postmenopause, which a woman is said to be in for the rest of her life.

The root cause of all of this is the hormonal response to what's known as "reproductive aging." Many hormones are at play, but primarily the female sex hormones—also known as the reproductive hormones—estrogen and progesterone.

> Note: It is essential to be aware that menopause can be triggered by a bi-lateral oophorectomy (removal of both ovaries), by treatment for cancers, and by use of estrogen-blocking drugs prescribed to people who have had estrogen receptor-positive (ER) cancers. Entering menopause suddenly is sometimes accompanied by more severe symptoms.

Hormones are messengers that help our cells understand what they need to do. Here let's look at the main players, and then how their changing status affects other hormones not associated with reproduction. Other variables are addressed throughout the book.

THE MAIN PLAYERS

Estrogen

Estrogen is like a vibrant party host—energetic, capable of great conversation, keeping everything organized, and also of having a great time. Estrogen is also thought to buffer brain and body against the effects of stress. When we have plenty of it, we can feel invincible.

Figure 1.1 will help you see how, though it is known as a reproductive hormone, estrogen has a bearing on our entire body, brain, and nervous system.

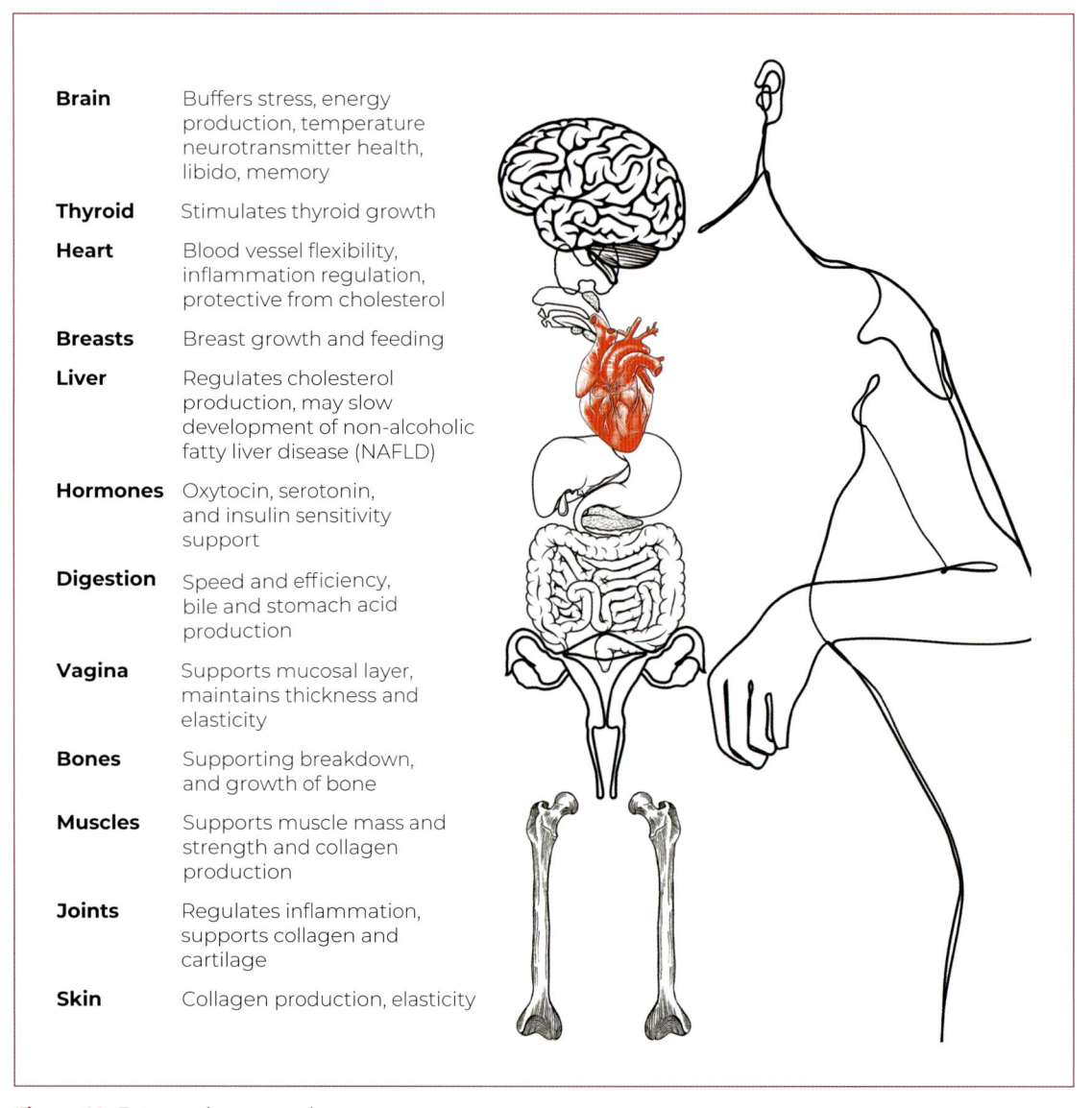

Brain	Buffers stress, energy production, temperature neurotransmitter health, libido, memory
Thyroid	Stimulates thyroid growth
Heart	Blood vessel flexibility, inflammation regulation, protective from cholesterol
Breasts	Breast growth and feeding
Liver	Regulates cholesterol production, may slow development of non-alcoholic fatty liver disease (NAFLD)
Hormones	Oxytocin, serotonin, and insulin sensitivity support
Digestion	Speed and efficiency, bile and stomach acid production
Vagina	Supports mucosal layer, maintains thickness and elasticity
Bones	Supporting breakdown, and growth of bone
Muscles	Supports muscle mass and strength and collagen production
Joints	Regulates inflammation, supports collagen and cartilage
Skin	Collagen production, elasticity

Figure 1.1 *Estrogen's many roles*

THE BIOCHEMISTRY OF MENOPAUSE   19

Progesterone

Progesterone aids sleep and calms us. We could see it as the kind aunt who we can all rely on for a hug and a gentle word to keep us calm in moments of stress, to bring us back to earth and give us a bowl of nourishing soup when we've overdone it!

Progesterone has a considerable effect on brain function and repair, and heart and breast health. It also aids sleep, is anti-depressant, is a sedative, aids cognition, helps normalize blood sugar, helps use fat for energy, and helps the growth of nervous system tissue.

Follicle-stimulating hormone

When the brain notices that the number of follicles in the ovaries is in decline as a woman approaches the end of her reproductive years, the hypothalamus signals the pituitary to produce more and more follicle-stimulating hormone (FSH). As FSH does its job and more follicles are ripened,

Hypothalamus
Pituitary

Estradiol and progesterone

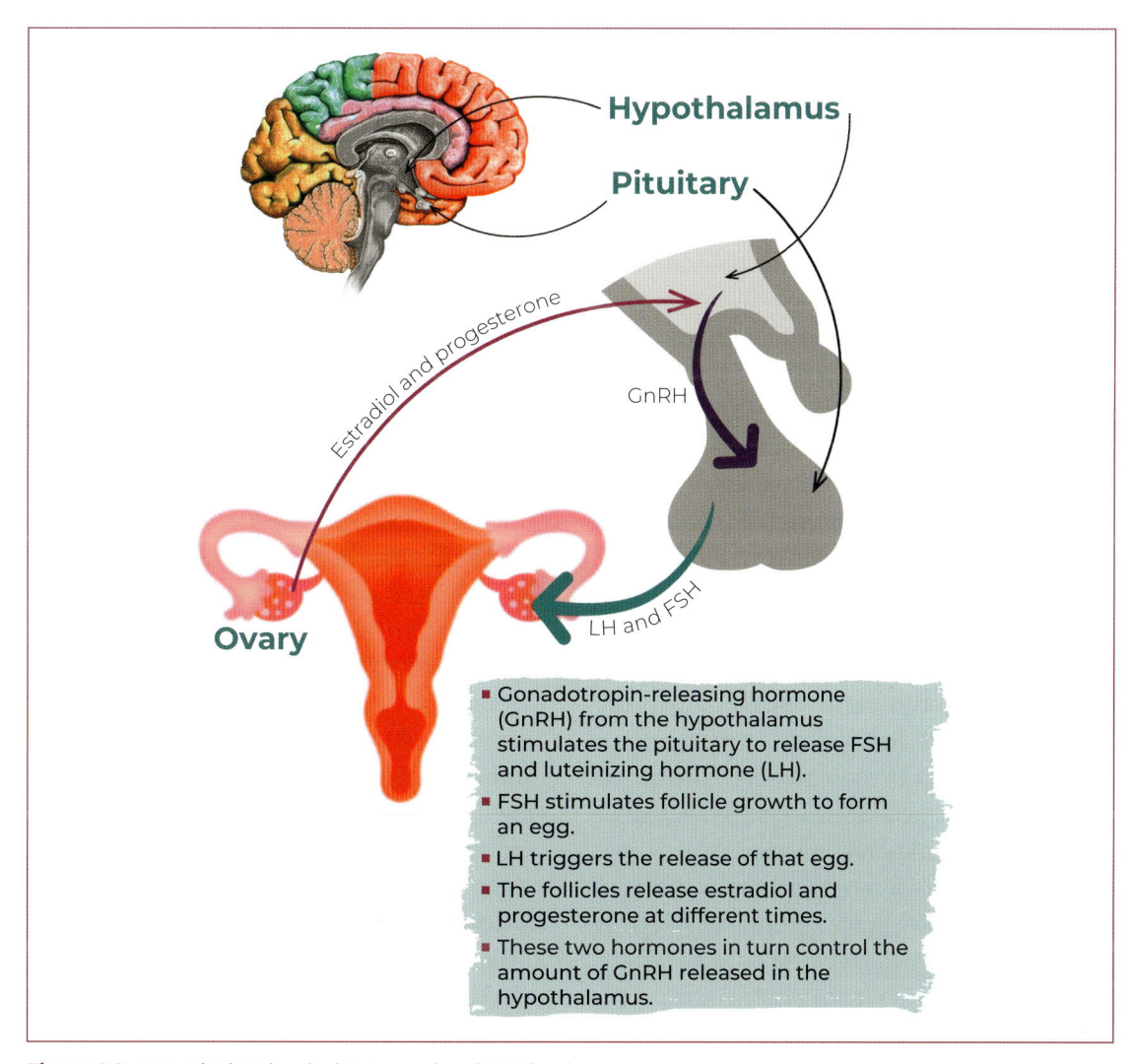

GnRH

Ovary

LH and FSH

- Gonadotropin-releasing hormone (GnRH) from the hypothalamus stimulates the pituitary to release FSH and luteinizing hormone (LH).
- FSH stimulates follicle growth to form an egg.
- LH triggers the release of that egg.
- The follicles release estradiol and progesterone at different times.
- These two hormones in turn control the amount of GnRH released in the hypothalamus.

Figure 1.2 *Hypothalamic-pituitary-ovarian (HPO) axis*

sometimes more than one egg is released simultaneously. This is one possible cause for the increased likelihood of fraternal twins later in a woman's life. FSH continues to increase after menopause.

In a normal monthly cycle, estrogen and progesterone are produced in the ovaries in response to signals from glands in the brain (the hypothalamic-pituitary-ovarian [HPO] axis), figure 1.2. FSH is produced by the pituitary gland to stimulate the ripening of a follicle to release an egg. After an egg is released, estrogen and progesterone are produced by the remaining follicle (corpus luteum). Estrogen dominates the first half of the cycle, progesterone the second. This creates the conditions for conception and pregnancy or menstrual bleeding, as appropriate.

THE SUPPORTING ROLES

Some of a woman's **testosterone** is produced in the ovaries. Its role is, among other things, intimately linked with reproductive functions, from libido to vaginal health. It is converted into estrogen, which is why women don't develop the male characteristics associated with it.

Cortisol is a necessary hormone, produced by the adrenal glands, levels of which normally rise in the morning and dwindle toward evening. It helps us to wake up and stay focused. It helps to regulate our blood sugar levels. When it dwindles as expected, the body can produce melatonin to support sleep. It is also produced at times of stress.

Melatonin, produced by the pineal gland, is a hormone that helps us fall asleep.

The gland responds to light levels, making melatonin more readily produced when we are exposed to evening light and darkness.

Oxytocin is a hormone which can be considered a reproductive hormone, given its role in labor and lactation, but also, you could say, because it helps women bond with their partner and offspring, two necessary attributes to aid successful procreation.

Serotonin is officially a neurotransmitter but is also referred to as a hormone. It supports mood, the brain, bones, digestion, and the production of melatonin.

Insulin, produced in the pancreas, helps to regulate blood glucose levels.

THE STAGES OF MENOPAUSE

There are distinct phases of the menopause, and distinct needs for each.

The late reproductive stage (LRS) and perimenopause

This little spoken-about phase is not recognized by most medical practitioners as being, essentially, part of perimenopause. But studies into it (Coslov et al, 2021; Cortes et al, 2023) have been analyzed, and the North American Menopause Society has made a statement about it. I expect it will be receiving more attention than it has had up to now, and I hope you will see why I believe it should.

As a woman comes toward the end of her reproductive years, usually around her late 30s or early 40s, her hormonal landscape begins to change, but periods are still pretty regular. It is a stage that can produce confusion and fear. Women may sense disconcerting symptoms, but because of regular bleeding, they often confuse it with illness and do not recognize it as the result of natural hormonal changes. So, for instance, if pre-menstrual syndrome (PMS) or pre-menstrual dysphoric disorder (PMDD) worsen, or she experiences some of the symptoms listed in the quote below, she may become concerned for her health.

> 'A recent scoping review of research about the LRS revealed **little attention to women's experiences during this stage**. Since 2001... only nine studies focused explicitly on the LRS. Results of these studies suggest that women reported **symptoms typically associated with the MT** [menopause transition] such as sleep disruption, hot flashes, breast pain, vaginal dryness, urinary incontinence and nocturia, memory and mood changes, and pain before their periods changed significantly.' (Coslov et al, 2021; my bold.)

Though women report the symptoms detailed in this quote, and additionally restlessness and anxiety, looking back on their 30s and early 40s, many women say they also experienced a variety of other changes. Anecdotally, in my work with hundreds of clients, I have seen these further experiences associated with this phase:

- Yearning to open a new chapter in work or home life
- Increased levels of energy and "going for it" in their exercise choices
- Increased libido
- Reduced libido
- Looking outside a committed relationship or noticing desire for new sexual connection
- Multitasking like a superhero
- Getting drunk more quickly and/or longer hangovers.

Some of the more positive of these traits can mean that women notice the difficult effects only in the background. 'I'm a bit sleepless, but I have boundless energy, so it seems okay;' 'I'm a little anxious, but I also feel confident and passionate about a new project, so it's not a problem.'

This phase segues into and overlaps with early perimenopause.

Perimenopause

Though "peri" means "around," medically perimenopause refers to the time leading up to menopause, and not, as the name suggests, the time either side of menopause. It is, however, an apt name because symptoms often continue after menopause.

Your students may notice, usually in their mid-40s, a number of struggles arising in their bodies (table 1.1). The journey from the LRS into the early stages of perimenopause occurs in a way that can't be narrowed down to a day. A fairly normal timeframe for the onset of symptomatic perimenopause is anywhere in a woman's 40s or early 50s.

For a woman in her mid-40s, a doctor will look for menstrual irregularity of plus or minus seven days and symptoms like hot flashes. For younger women, further investigation would be carried out.

The symptomatic time can be anything from a few months to many years, with the North American Menopause Society determining the duration as between four and eight years (Menopause 101: A primer for the perimenopausal).

Table 1.1 *Some symptoms of the perimenopause*

Common	Less common
Hot flashes (flushes)	Breast pain
Fatigue	Nausea
Low mood	Itchy skin
Anxiety	Digestive issues
Sleep disturbance	Urinary infections
Change of libido	Dizziness (vertigo)
Acopia/overwhelm	Bladder weakness
Irregular periods	Allergies
Heavy/light bleeds	Gum issues
Brain fog	Tingling extremities
Concentration loss	Electric shocks
Weight gain	Burning tongue
Vaginal dryness	Tinnitus
Increased PMT	Brittle nails
Irritability	Hair loss
Night sweats	Changing body odor
Headaches/migraines	Palpitations
	Panic attacks

Table 1.1 could be changed on a regular basis, depending on who you talk to, with more and more issues being blamed on menopause when things may not necessarily be so simple. I have encountered many estimates for numbers of symptoms, from 34 upward. Research suggests that:

- Roughly 20% of women sail through perimenopause with very few, and very mild symptoms.
- Roughly 60% have a journey marked by more numerous and/or more-or-less intense symptoms that come and go. They can be upsetting, affecting their physical, mental, and emotional comfort and resilience in everyday situations. Of course, within this 60% there is a spectrum of experience.
- Roughly 20% experience symptoms to a degree of intensity that limits their ability to live their lives as they used to, and seriously affects their physical, mental, and/or emotional health, potentially to a disabling level.

Perimenopause usually occurs naturally with the decline of ovarian follicles. With any change in menstruation or ovulation, however slight, there are changes in hormone levels (figure 1.3). However,

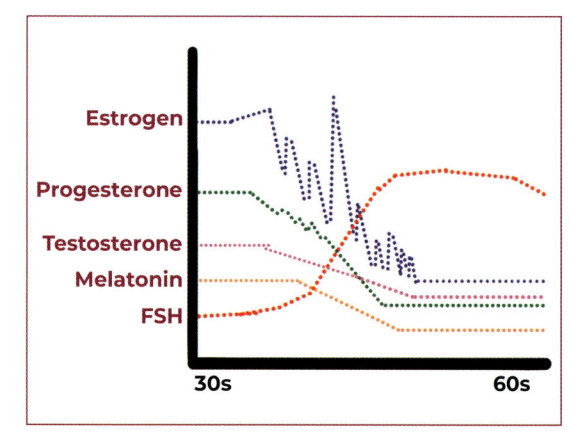

Figure 1.3 *Unpredictable menopause graph*

though most women think of the stages of menopause as being about loss of hormones, symptoms of the LRS, and indeed perimenopause, are decidedly not just about decrease of estrogen—which can even increase (Santoro, 1996)—and involve other hormones.

You will notice in figure 1.3 that progesterone has a smoother decline than estrogen and begins to drop sooner, but please note that this graph does not purport to be precise. I made it myself, with no measuring tape or scientific instruments, specifically because there is such wildly fluctuating biochemistry that a graph that suggests anything more specific might lead you to expect some predictability!

Biochemically, symptoms may be due, at different times, to:

- Reduced progesterone
- Increased estrogen
- Decreased estrogen
- Increased cortisol
- Decreased testosterone
- Increased blood sugar peaks and troughs
- Increased follicle-stimulating hormone.

Less-studied changes in melatonin, serotonin, and oxytocin can also contribute.

Reduced progesterone and melatonin both contribute to sleep issues. Reduced testosterone can result in lower energy, lower libido, difficulty reaching orgasm, fatigue, concentration issues, muscular weakness, bone loss, thinning hair, and reduced vaginal lubrication. Increased FSH can cause hot flashes, weight gain, vaginal dryness, sleep issues, and bone loss. Estrogen and progesterone support insulin sensitivity, which is how we avoid the blood sugar imbalance that can exacerbate symptoms. Serotonin and oxytocin levels are known to decrease, potentially contributing to depression, low melatonin, digestive issues, lack of joy, impatience with family, and relationship struggles. Increased and/or dysregulated cortisol can result in sleeplessness, anxiety, weight gain, osteoporosis, and more.

> No intervention other than hormone therapy can increase the levels of the three reproductive hormones (estrogen, progesterone, and testosterone) in a woman's body once she has entered perimenopause. By hormone therapy I mean what is often called menopause hormone therapy (MHT) or hormone replacement therapy (HRT). I shall be using MHT as shorthand in this book.

Estrogen dominance, or unopposed estrogen (when progesterone is lower in relation to estrogen than hitherto), is not universal, and its relevance to perimenopause is debated. But if it is present, it produces symptoms all of its own, like sleeplessness, tender breasts, increased PMT, bloating, anxiety, and more.

As you can see from figure 1.3, estrogen in particular doesn't decline in a linear fashion, but fluctuates unpredictably. This is why perimenopause can be characterized by weeks or months when a woman thinks it's all over, the symptoms have abated, only to find a resurgence of some previous symptoms, or new ones, for another period of weeks or months.

When you look at the list of symptoms, you may wonder why there are such wide and varied effects. Aside from what you have already read above, this is also because there are estrogen and progesterone receptors on many tissue cells throughout the body. A receptor is like a little flag, exactly shaped to receive the hormone it needs to help it fulfil its role.

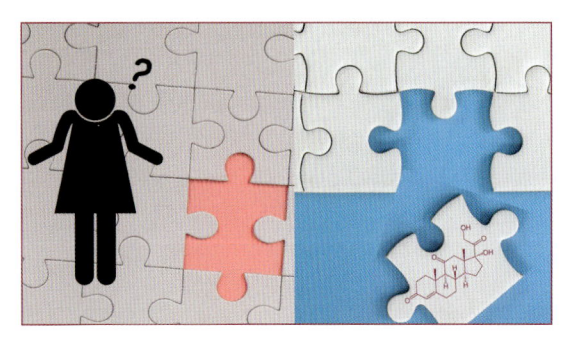

Figure 1.4 *An estrogen molecule fits perfectly into this "cell," to let it know what to do to fulfil its purpose*

Just like a jigsaw piece, the hormone will only fit in its perfect docking station (figure 1.4). Without the passing hormones the cells are left wondering what their job is, so you can begin to understand the confusion in the body. These receptors are found in areas of the brain that affect mood, in the pelvic floor and even the bladder, the vagina, the skin, vascular tissue, and in the gut. The list goes on. And on.

Considering that there are so many biochemical variables, even before we take health status and life-load into account, we see the folly of trying to find exact reasons why our students are struggling, and instead address that which may help in many scenarios.

> Throughout life, low levels of estrogen can occur from excessive exercising, excessive dieting, or from medical treatments like radiotherapy and chemotherapy, with symptoms similar to perimenopause.

Postmenopause

Menopause is that one day, often much anticipated, when a woman has had no menstrual bleeding for 12 consecutive months. The rest of your life is said to be postmenopausal.

Reaching menopause between 40 and 45 would be considered natural but early. After 45 would not be considered abnormal. There is a growing number of women being diagnosed with premature ovarian insufficiency (POI) which is when menopause is reached early, even as early as the teenage years, but anything up to around 40.

After menopause, FSH levels can be high but will usually gradually fall and stabilize. Women continue to produce some progesterone and estrone (a type of estrogen). Postmenopausally, these sex hormones are produced in small amounts in the ovaries and the adrenal glands, and estrone is also produced in adipose tissue (fat).

Some women find that symptoms decrease and disappear, some find they continue for a time, and some find some aspects linger for many years. There are a few theories, but in reality we don't know why many women's perimenopause symptoms dissipate. The good news is that, for the vast majority, the storm subsides and calmer conditions prevail, sometimes even calmer than before.

THE HEALTH IMPLICATIONS OF MENOPAUSE

The symptoms of perimenopause are not, in themselves, a risk to life. It is not an illness. Symptoms are quite separate from what are sometimes known as the health concerns of menopause. Essentially, menopause marks an increase in risk to the health of certain areas.

There are changes to a woman's level of health risk whenever or however she enters menopause. It is immensely important to take them into account to avoid causing your students harm in the present, and to support them for the future. These changes come to men also, but as a result of biological rather than reproductive aging, but for women the risks of osteoporosis and dementia will, unfortunately, always be higher.

The three main recognized increased health risks of menopause are:

- Osteoporosis
- Cardiovascular disease
- Cognitive decline.

Osteoporosis may begin now because, for example:

- From our 30s onward, the rate of bone building reduces and that of breakdown increases.
- In the five or so years postmenopause, bone loss accelerates further.
- Muscle mass reduces, leading to less robust stimulus to the bones.
- Fatigue can impact the ability to do appropriate exercise.
- The digestive system may become less efficient at absorption of essential minerals and vitamins needed to maintain bone mineral density (BMD).

Cardiovascular disease becomes a concern for a number of reasons, including:

- Cholesterol levels seem to rise in women around this time, which may be because of lifestyle factors or a consequence of other effects of perimenopause, but the causes are not certain.
- Estrogen has a positive effect on the flexibility of blood vessels in the heart, keeping them mobile and supple in younger women. Without this, the potential for build-up of plaque in usually mobile pathways may increase.
- Estrogen can be abrasive of the arterial walls in older women (which is one reason why MHT becomes less safe as women age).
- The likelihood of high blood pressure can increase in later perimenopause and postmenopause, in part because progesterone has diuretic effects.

Cognitive decline becomes a concern owing largely to reduced levels of estrogen which, among other benefits:

- has a buffering effect on the effects of stress on the brain.

- is key for energy production in the brain. It pushes nerves to burn glucose to make energy.
- has a role to play in the health of our neurotransmitters.

In addition, research is showing that amyloid plaques (which are unusual collections of otherwise normal proteins that build up in the brain, potentially damaging neurons) increase by about 20% in the brains of some perimenopausal women (mostly those with the APOE4 gene). Note that amyloid plaques can be present in the brains of people who never develop Alzheimer's disease. They are only one risk-factor for Alzheimer's disease, and their presence does not mean that the disease is inevitable.

There are other areas potentially impacted by menopause. These include:

- Pelvic floor
- Genitourinary system
- Joints
- Blood sugar regulation
- Liver function
- Lung function
- Lymphatic system
- Digestion
- Emotional health
- Thyroid health.

Supporting these concerns is dealt with in chapters 4 and 5. Two are not directly dealt with in further chapters, so I explain them briefly below.

Thyroid health

This is not directly affected by perimenopause, but thyroid function needs to be monitored for a number of reasons.

- Symptoms of both hypo- and hyperthyroidism are shared with symptoms of perimenopause, so it may be easy to ignore thyroid issues if women assume that all their symptoms are directly because of menopause.
- If a woman with hypothyroid starts oral MHT, her thyroid medications may need adjusting.
- Thyroid issues are hugely more common in women than in men, and can begin in midlife, though not as a direct result of perimenopause. A mixture of issues may be causing problems. Getting hypo- or hyperthyroidism treated may relieve some women of symptoms that she thought were perimenopausal.
- It is also possible that, when treated, the symptoms that are attributable to perimenopause may lessen as thyroid issues can exacerbate symptoms.

Thyroid dysfunction is a condition that necessitates medical support.

Lung function

This can be impaired and/or lung capacity reduced. Research into this is not wide, but it does seem to begin in perimenopause and to continue thereafter (Triebner et al, 2016). Reasons have not been fully established, but it is thought it may be related to increased inflammation. Impaired lung function can be one of the reasons for greater fatigue after exercise. It is important to continue to perform exercise that challenges the lungs, but not to push to the point of feeling symptoms of oxygen lack, like dizziness and shortness of breath. Pranayama can improve lung function.

THE ROLE OF STRESS

The human body is designed to experience stress and react to it. It's part of our survival mechanism. When we are under threat, the hypothalamus-pituitary-adrenal (HPA) axis creates the conditions for the release of adrenaline and cortisol into the system.

At the same time, a calming neurotransmitter called GABA decreases (figure 1.5). This is acute stress, and is positive when we need to run from danger or meet an important deadline; it keeps us alert and ready. It is perfectly healthy and functional as long our nervous system is able to return to rest mode after the stressor has passed.

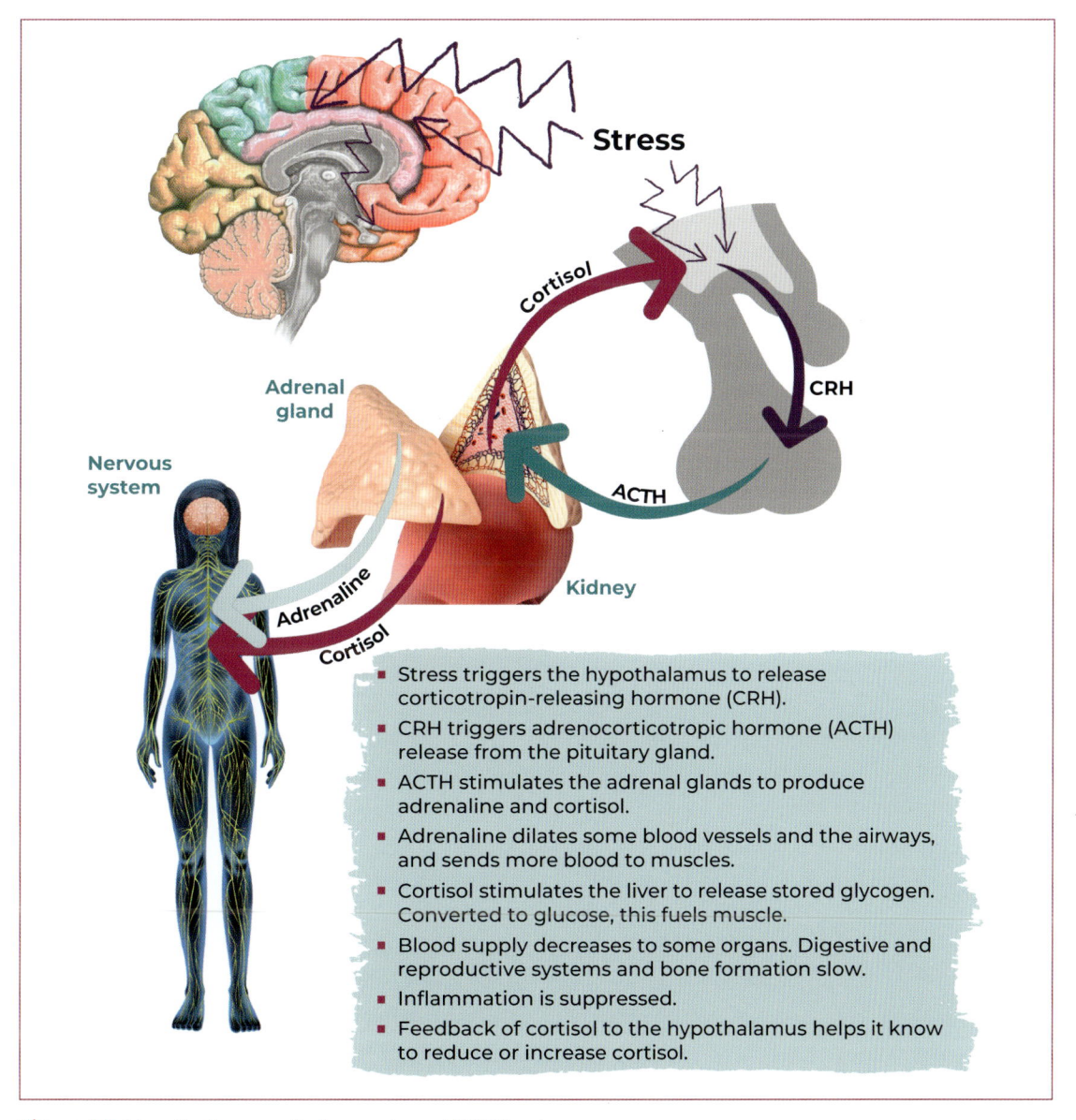

- Stress triggers the hypothalamus to release corticotropin-releasing hormone (CRH).
- CRH triggers adrenocorticotropic hormone (ACTH) release from the pituitary gland.
- ACTH stimulates the adrenal glands to produce adrenaline and cortisol.
- Adrenaline dilates some blood vessels and the airways, and sends more blood to muscles.
- Cortisol stimulates the liver to release stored glycogen. Converted to glucose, this fuels muscle.
- Blood supply decreases to some organs. Digestive and reproductive systems and bone formation slow.
- Inflammation is suppressed.
- Feedback of cortisol to the hypothalamus helps it know to reduce or increase cortisol.

Figure 1.5 *Hypothalamus-pituitary-adrenal (HPA) axis*

The accumulation of burdens that challenge resilience and health at any time is known as our allostatic load. Stress becomes negative ("distress") or chronic when a person faces continuous challenges without relief or relaxation between challenges, or without awareness of when the stressor will end. That last phrase is significant. You can see that the lack of certainty around even just the duration of perimenopause could be a chronic stress, adding to that allostatic load.

Stress can also increase as the changing levels of hormones in perimenopause cause changes in the efficiency and health of neurotransmitters (molecules that enable signaling throughout the body). Potentially, as in the reduced toleration of temperature variation that contributes to hot flashes, this can alter the range of stressors women can manage with equilibrium (figure 1.6).

So women in perimenopause may be more likely to react as if on a "hair trigger," as many women will attest, describing themselves as impatient and quick to feel overwhelmed. This perceived inability to cope with life can lead to a constant underlying—or even overt—state of fear. This may create a long-term stress response which in turn exacerbates the hair-trigger tendency, in addition to exacerbating the perimenopause symptoms like sleeplessness, anxiety, and hot flashes. A vicious circle ensues.

What's interesting in figure 1.6 is the number of symptoms which are the same as the symptoms of perimenopause.

> 'The long-term activation of the stress response system and the overexposure to cortisol and other stress hormones ... can disrupt almost all your body's processes. This puts you at increased risk of many health problems, including: anxiety, depression, digestive problems, headaches, muscle tension and pain, heart disease, heart attack, high blood pressure and stroke, sleep problems, weight gain, memory and concentration impairment.' (Mayo Clinic, 2021)

They also mirror the health concerns of menopause like higher cholesterol and lower bone density.

Does this mean that these symptoms and health concerns are not connected with the changing levels of the sex hormones? No. But it indicates that any stressor, whether it's a body dealing with huge change or allostatic load of any sort, can result in symptoms. What I am illustrating here is the fact that we can

Brain
brain fog, concentration issues, low libido depression, anxiety, irritability, sleep disturbance, headaches, dizziness

Cardiovascular (CV)
higher cholesterol and blood pressure, palpitations, increased risk of CV events

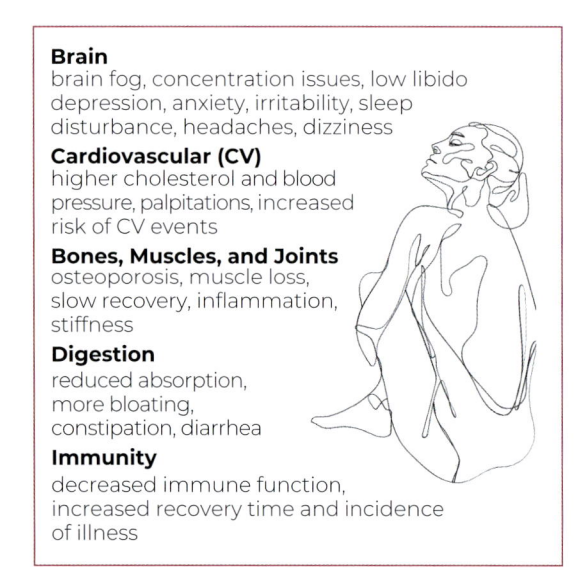

Bones, Muscles, and Joints
osteoporosis, muscle loss, slow recovery, inflammation, stiffness

Digestion
reduced absorption, more bloating, constipation, diarrhea

Immunity
decreased immune function, increased recovery time and incidence of illness

Figure 1.6 *Some effects of chronic stress*

never be sure what the cause of pretty much anything is!

Some symptoms may disappear when we look after our nervous system or make changes to support physical health. When these have been cared for, we can be (almost) certain that what remains is because of the reduction of the sex hormones, and not because of life-load or health challenges. This may make a woman's choices for self-care, particularly regarding medical intervention, clearer.

Along with the potential to reduce symptoms, reducing stressors, and learning to return to a state of ease after stress may also support future health, in particular the three main areas that are known to be affected by menopause: the bones, the heart, and the brain.

The information in this chapter is a lot to take in, and your students don't need to know all of it, not least because of the stress it may induce. Be assured that from your reading so far, you are already more informed than the vast majority of your students, and more equipped to help.

Sharing this information sensitively, and sometimes sparingly, will go a long way to supporting them.

Anecdotally, in my own observations from working with them:

- Women who are already suffering from stress before perimenopause (say a stressful job, a bereavement, a difficult relationship, a health scare) tend to have a more symptomatic journey.
- Women who are unaware of what is going on in their bodies, or what to expect, have a more difficult journey.
- Women who resist acknowledging what is occurring, or are resistant to or frightened of the changes, tend to have a more difficult journey.
- Once women become informed, and are then helped to come toward acceptance, their struggles seem to lighten. The symptoms remain, but the attendant stress is eased; in turn, the symptoms become less intense or intrusive, and potentially the woman is enabled to separate the symptoms from the external life-struggles.

CHAPTER 2
RESEARCH INTO YOGA FOR MENOPAUSE

The more I looked into scientific research into what eases the perimenopause experience and protects future health outside of yoga, the more I realized how the ancient yogis intuited a great deal when developing some of yoga's elements, without the benefits of the scientific knowledge of human systems that we have now.

But Western science is an excellent tool for proving efficacy and safety. After plentiful blunders over the centuries, it is more and more evident that we need to care for health and wellbeing in ways that are *known* to be of benefit, and to avoid harm. So, while trusting much of the tradition of yoga, I ask for more than just trust, especially since yoga in the West is far removed from what it was a thousand years ago, and people are prey to modern pressures to achieve that may not support women's real needs.

THE EVIDENCE FOR YOGA

Having read the last chapter, your mind may be starting to connect the dots between the many issues that arise in menopause and how you might support them, given what you already believe to be the benefits of yoga for the health and wellbeing of the general population. Indeed, there is plenty of research that provides evidence of many of those benefits.

However, though there are studies of yoga's benefits specifically for people in peri- and post-menopause, these are comparatively few. Some are positive (Cramer et al, 2018); some seem to contradict those positives (Lee et al, 2009). The vast majority of these studies are explorations of whether yoga *as we already know it* can help with symptoms, rather than of yoga *adjusted* and *targeted* toward the changes brought on by peri- and post-menopause.

At the time of writing, there is only one study I have managed to find that is somewhat more specific. It researched a cohort of women given yoga practices to do, twinned with 'the information support method.' This information included positive psychological "hints," education about menopause, and individualized recommendations (Lu et al, 2020). This is closer to my reimagining of yoga to serve menopausal needs. Results were promising, but I cannot, as yet, find any robustly researched yoga protocol that is steered toward menopause, both through information *and* specific practices, as I offer in this book and in my teacher training.

You may have read articles that quote studies, or perhaps read the conclusions of some studies. They may appear more encouraging than I seem to imply here. Indeed, there are many great studies listed in the bibliography for you to read. But I'm sure you're aware that reading studies is a nuanced job that requires a statistician's mind, among other skills. I have been nursed through reading research by a colleague who has these skills, and though I am better at it than I was, I still have to hold myself back from delighting in what at first glance seems like a fabulous result that supports what I would like to be true.

For example, there was a study into the benefits of yoga in reducing perimenopause symptoms for women who had begun practicing yoga before menopause (Souza et al, 2022). The results were really encouraging: almost 40% of the practitioners had no menopause symptoms, and none had severe symptoms. Compared with the two other groups studied (control groups who were not doing yoga: one group doing physical activity like weight training and/or aerobic exercise, and one sedentary group), the yogis were experiencing less menopausal discomfort in all areas. So, this tells us that practicing yoga before menopause may lead to a less intense perimenopause experience.

That's a nice result for some long-term practitioners (most of whom were teachers), but it doesn't tell us that yoga is an effective intervention for newcomers. Given that many women in need of additional or alternative support for their symptoms may only recognize this need when hormonal changes and symptoms have already begun, and may therefore not be regular practitioners, this study is not, to my mind, directly applicable to what I think yoga could be to women in the MT and beyond.

In addition, reading past the abstract (a summary of the study, its methods, and its outcomes), we see that most of the yoga group had already been practicing yoga (mostly *one* style) on average five times per week for about 12 years, were also non-smokers who did not use alcohol, were more likely to eat healthily, and were in sexually active relationships (all known contributors to health and wellbeing). The authors point out that these may be factors that explain the difference between the yoga and control groups. In addition, in the measuring scales they used, the results in two incredibly important areas (hot flashes and insomnia) varied from *significant* in one scale to *not significant* in the other.

Despite all these issues, I see this study cited in articles talking about yoga's benefits for menopause without these essential pieces of information, suggesting women take up yoga to manage their menopause. Because, although the authors responsibly conclude, 'Climacteric women who had started to practice yoga in premenopause and had already practiced it for at least five years had a low frequency and intensity of climacteric symptoms and good quality of life. Results were more expressive compared to sedentary women'

(Souza et al, 2022, p.5), what I believe we can truly say about this study is that some long-term committed practitioners of yoga, most of whom did not smoke or take alcohol and had a healthy diet, suffered fewer symptoms than a sedentary group, and had slightly better results than a group who were physically active.

This is good news of course, because even slight improvement is valuable. In fact, we could even claim that some of the contributory factors like a healthy lifestyle are, in a way, part of yoga's principles and encouraged in the teachings. But not every yoga student does more than just one class a week, or dives so deeply into it as a lifestyle as this small group of (mostly) experienced yoga teachers.

Unfortunately these results are not likely to encourage healthcare professionals to recommend yoga for the relief of symptoms, because despite how a teacher may interpret them and write about them, they provide no proof that it does so. I would like to see yoga teachers do what we can to encourage yoga to become a recommended intervention in the medical world and trusted menopause societies, as I think it could be. So if you choose to quote it, please do so responsibly (which may mean you need to purchase the study which, at the time of writing, is behind a paywall).

I would absolutely recommend yoga to help with our experience of many symptoms because it can greatly calm the resistance and/or negative reactions that can add so dramatically to the intensity of the storm. I think all yoga practitioners experience that calming with regard to all life challenges, but none of us would imagine this is a result of one pose or sequence, but a whole practice. In fact, **there is no research to suggest that any one pose benefits any particular symptom or health concern of perimenopause or postmenopause.**

Yet we see claims about individual poses made—in articles and by teachers—again and again, not just regarding menopause. Whose fault is it? Many of these claims have been made for decades, even centuries, and handed down in a guru-style tradition where questioning the teachings is not on offer. A teacher may then take what they have been told and disseminate it further. In a faith-based system, she is being a faithful yoga teacher. Many individual claims about some specific yoga postures or practices, made when yoga was barely researched at all, have become the yogic equivalent of an urban myth. In fact, in her years of poring over vast amounts of research, Dr Mary Flaherty found evidence for specific benefits attributed to an individual asana to be convincing for only *one* posture.

As teachers, as well as wanting to trust and uphold what we have learnt in training, we may also feel pressure to make promises, to have answers, and to offer certainties, because the world demands that now. When we mix unthinking claims with a culture that wants quick fixes, this trend of perhaps overselling yoga's benefits will only grow.

In reality, there is no intervention (even evidence-based medical treatment) guaranteed to help every individual.

I cannot adequately express how important I feel it is to be careful about what we claim. Women are being promised so much at a time when they need so much. Citing a study like the one above in an effort to promote yoga for menopause to the general population is to add to the barrage of false promises women are navigating in wellness culture, at a vulnerable time in their lives.

If we as teachers make promises based on no evidence, irrelevant or scant evidence (even if more research may eventually prove something true that we don't currently know), we may, at best, disappoint our students and be ourselves vulnerable to accusations of making false claims. At worst, we may cause women who come to us to try to achieve relief through our suggestions to judge *themselves* as lacking when such interventions fail to meet their expectations.

Many women's bodies are more vulnerable in perimenopause and postmenopause, and so is their mental health and self-esteem. Complex postures may be more likely to injure, and being unable to "achieve" certain shapes or even complex breath work may shatter already impoverished self-esteem, and injury or low mood can lead to loss of movement potential or inclination. This is the opposite of supporting menopausal needs!

Could we even fail to protect women from injury? I believe so. Though there is research into yoga that shows a variety of results for the improvement of vasomotor symptoms (the collective term for hot flashes and night sweats), more positive results come unfortunately from less-than-optimal studies. More robust studies show results from "did not improve" (Newton et al, 2014) to improvements that were "comparable to exercise" (Cramer et al, 2018), with a more reasonable overall conclusion that yoga improves the experience, but not the duration or frequency (Flaherty, 2020). Yet, if a woman Googles "yoga for hot flashes" and in her need tries some of the postures that pop up, she may do herself damage.

The following are some examples of dubious and potentially injurious claims I have seen:

- **Head-to-knee forward bend 'helps symptoms of menopause.'** There is no evidence for this. In addition, women are more likely to have osteopenia or osteoporosis than in premenopause so this pose would be contraindicated; it can also be hard on changed and challenged cartilage, fascia, soft tissue, and joints.
- **Shoulder stand 'relieves symptoms of menopause.'** Again, no evidence. It is also a risky pose to be in and to exit, and difficult to achieve. In addition, the neck position, especially with the added weight of the body above it, has serious contraindications for osteoporosis.
- **Reclining cobbler 'relieves symptoms of menopause and stress.'** There is no evidence of either for the pose in isolation. You will discover on p.90 that I am a huge fan of this pose. But the benefits may be as much from what you do while in the pose, and even from just stopping and taking the time to

do it. My time in this pose helped me immensely through my perimenopause, and helped me to be more able to handle the second half of my day because I was no longer depleted. But a nap or meditation or rest or deep breathing in any pleasant restorative pose, or *any* activity that supports the nervous system could have been just as helpful. In fact, I would often fall asleep in this pose, and that nap could have been the main reason it helped me.

- **Downward dog 'helps reduce osteoporosis.'** There is no convincing study that gives us any such assurance about this pose in isolation. So much more needs to be done than just making this shape, or any shape! This pose was included in a study which showed benefits for osteoporosis, but even if this particular study had been run with a more solid methodology, the pose on its own has not been studied. The irresponsibility of this claim worries me, as it encourages women to look for easy ways to do things like reverse osteoporosis. What is needed to reduce osteoporosis is considerable, from bearing heavy weight, to nutrition and more. No number of downward dogs is going to give the benefits a woman might hope for after a diagnosis of low bone mass.
- **Pose dedicated to the sage Marichi has 'a therapeutic application for obesity.'** Leaving aside the fact that twists, especially bound twists, are risky for those with low bone density in the spine, this claim is exceptionally simplistic and inflated. I would suggest you look at this claim and ask yourself what it even means, or if indeed it means anything at all. Many variations of this pose are contraindicated for osteoporosis.

Do I seem hard on yoga? It is not my intention. My intention in this chapter is to say what troubles me, then put it aside and set us up for an **evidence-based reimagining**. These terms may seem to contradict each other, one pragmatic, the other creative. But it is upon a bedrock of certainty that we can let our imaginations create new possibilities. Indeed, all science is based on an imagining that someone then sets about analyzing to see if it was true.

I dissected the study above, and the poses above as recommended in an online article, only as examples of how headlines from studies or articles are often grabbed and used without further examination. But in fact I have very little doubt that a regular yoga practice, and even cherry-picking a few elements to practice regularly, can lessen the intensity and possibly even the number of perimenopause symptoms and protect, as far as it's possible to do so, future health. It is certainly better than doing nothing to support overall wellbeing.

I can't be at all certain that yoga is more beneficial than exercise. But my instinct tells me it should be, or could be, given that it also addresses nervous system regulation, spiritual connection, intelligent inquiry, empathetic connection, and even nutrition (in its encouragement toward eating calming, pure foods), all of which have known health benefits and are not part of most exercise regimes.

But at the moment, it is not okay for me to say other than that yoga includes these factors, and that these factors support health, and to say that some of them are also are known to reduce the intensity of some menopause symptoms. We can use language to encourage people toward yoga for menopause to see if it works for them individually, but we cannot make promises, not least because, unless someone enters into a long-term committed yoga journey, they are unlikely to take up all its tenets.

My hope is that women who come to my weekly classes will benefit without having to devote themselves to a massive change in lifestyle, given that most of our students have demands in life at this stage that may make a full commitment to yoga unachievable. I expect these are the kinds of women most of you reading this book tend to have in your classes too.

Of course, science doesn't have all the answers. But at a time when women can be desperate for solutions, we must *know* that what we are claiming is true. We should be sure that what we are offering is truly valuable, at least for most people, rather than hope or guess, or worse, repeat what someone else has claimed. Until we know more. What we *do* know is not headline-grabbing, but avoiding uncertain claims is to approach our students truthfully. Satya.

Is this evidence enough?

Given all we do know about yoga, it is hard to understand why the most glowing recommendations you'll see from the medical community are the likes of 'may be helpful, but more research is needed,' especially because we know yoga helps us manage stress, helps keep muscles strong, reduces anxiety, and aches and pains. Also, elements of it are akin to well-established menopause supports like "paced breathing" and cognitive behavioral therapy (CBT).

Partly this is because of the less-than-conclusive research I have just spoken about, and also because there have not been as many studies into how yoga can relieve menopause struggles as have been conducted into yoga for other issues (or as there have been into pharmaceuticals, exercise, and nutrition, of course). In addition, because yoga is such a broad tradition, with so many elements, creative teachers, and styles, it is notoriously difficult to produce repeatable clinical studies showing its benefits.

The medical profession require repeatable and repeated studies with the same outcomes to be able to recommend something. So if you see someone in the medical profession advising a lifestyle practice, it is likely because there is an abundance of peer-reviewed, statistically significant research for them to feel comfortable doing that.

To get to a really reliable, research-based protocol for menopause relief and health protection through yoga, it would probably have to be so tediously repetitive and scripted to avoid variation that the richness and joy of yoga would be lost for the sake of a statistically significant repeated outcome! So we may need to content ourselves with taking a backseat to medicine, Pilates, CBT, and other more widely recommended supports.

Thankfully, research is plentiful and convincing enough to enable us to say:

- Yoga supports sleep in most (Wang et al, 2020).
- Yoga can reduce stress (Shohani et al, 2018; Shobana et al, 2022).
- It can reduce cortisol levels (Thirthalli et al, 2013).
- Yoga nidra helps reduce anxiety (Ferreira-Vorkapic et al, 2018).
- Pranayama can support cardiovascular health (Saoji et al, 2019).
- Yoga supports brain health and structure in many ways (van Aalst et al, 2020).
- It can reduce inflammation (Djalilova et al, 2018) and improve immunity (Falkenberg et al, 2018).
- It improves balance (Kadachha et al, 2016).
- Yoga seems to increase beneficial neurotransmitters like serotonin and GABA (Streeter et al, 2010; Kjaer et al, 2002).
- It improves interoception (which was seen to reduce risk of burnout) (Heeter et al, 2021).
- We know it may help increase or preserve the length of telomeres (the parts of our chromosomes whose shortening is associated with aging) (Krishna et al, 2015).
- It can reduce oxidative stress associated with aging (Krishna et al, 2015; Tolahunase et al, 2017).
- It helps improve strength (Madanmohan et al, 1992).
- It helps relieve depression (Streeter et al, 2017; Bridges & Sharma, 2017).
- It can improve heartrate variability (Lin et al, 2015).
- It can reduce risk of developing type 2 diabetes (Kaur et al, 2021).
- It can reduce pain levels in some areas and/or conditions (NCCIH, 2020).

There are thousands of studies that could be listed here. If you want to find out more, I recommend the book *Does Yoga Work? Answers from Science* by Mary Flaherty PhD.

Most positives associated with yoga are seen where it includes asana, pranayama, and meditation together (Flaherty, 2020). There are a few exceptions. For instance, there is robust evidence that Kirtan Kriya can be an aid to cognitive function for people in the early stages of Alzheimer's disease (Innes et al, 2018), which given some of the health concerns of menopause makes this a worthwhile practice to consider. Research is still ongoing, however, as to whether this is because of the focus required to perform it, because of the movement of the tongue, or because of the meaning of the sounds (what are the results for people who understand the Sanskrit versus those who don't?) etcetera, and begs the question whether a similar made-up practice that requires digital, oral, verbal, and mental elements might work just as well.

Kapalabhati has been shown to be of some benefit for pelvic floor strength and reduction of urinary leakage in menopausal women (Patil & Honkalas, 2022), and another study showed its benefits for heart rate variability, which supports the possibility that it can aid autonomic nervous system regulation (Malhotra et al, 2022). This study was done on regular practitioners, not beginners, and you can imagine that it could take some time to achieve a level of precision and correct practice for beginners.

A study into bhastrika shows benefit for lung function (Budhi et al, 2019), though this study was done on young males, who of course would have a very different reaction to exertion from that of women in the stages of menopause.

You will often see kapalabhati and bhastrika listed as pranayama to avoid in perimenopause. In Chapter 3 f), you will see why I believe this may be unnecessary. Conversely, you will often see sitali and sitkari breath recommended. They can be very pleasant. However, I don't appreciate repeated claims I see in almost every article on using yoga for menopause symptoms that these practices can reduce the frequency or severity of hot flashes, as we do not have any such evidence. These claims are based on the assumption that these practices reduce body temperature, but to date I cannot find evidence of this. Even if it did reduce temperature, having a hot body is only one of very many triggers, and is not always a trigger—if it was, you would never see a perimenopausal woman heading off on a sun holiday! Once a hot flash starts, it will run its course, because, though it may be wrong, your brain thinks the flash is imperative for your safety, to stop you overheating. If you have ever had a flash outdoors on a cold day, you will know that cool air entering your mouth and lungs, though it may feel nice, doesn't stop or lessen it!

In addition to focusing on specific elements within yoga that have researched benefits relevant to this life stage, teaching Yoga for Menopause and Beyond benefits from the addition of techniques cherry-picked from a wide variety of reliable studies from outside yoga, including:

- CBT (Norton, 2014) is a commonly recommended tool which is very similar to the yoga principles of *svadhyaya* (self-study: what exactly is occurring in me and in my environment?), *satya* (truth, i.e., letting go of creating a story that is exaggerated/not true or catastrophizing), *pratipaksha-bhavana* (which translates as "opposite sentiment," a positive intervention for negative thinking), and *ahimsa* (do no harm—in this case, via self-damaging negative thinking or catastrophizing).
- There are some really achievable breathing practices, similar to pranayama detailed in Chapter 3 (Sood et al, 2013; Zaied et al, 2021).
- Strength measures very similar to bandhas (energetic locks) are part of a fairly new exercise protocol for PF health called "hypopressive training." All of these yoga-style (but not officially yoga!) tools will be detailed in further chapters.

SELLING YOGA FOR MENOPAUSE

In addition to avoiding claims of which you are unsure, I ask you to avoid trying to get people into your classes by the induction of fear. Phrases like 'estrogen deficient' or suggestions that 'if you don't keep moving your health will suffer' are not supportive to women, who are often very worried. Our main job is to soothe, and then, if women come to our classes, to support.

I would ask you also to be mindful about what you say is necessary for health. For instance, I recently saw in a post on social media a quote from Joseph Pilates: 'If your spine is inflexibly stiff at 30, you are old. If it is completely flexible at 60, you are young.' The question in the post was 'How old are you?' and the post showed the teacher moving in and out of child's pose and a very extended cobra. Before reading on, can you consider how this might be an unhelpful post for a perimenopausal cohort, or indeed for the entire population?

My thoughts are that, though it was genuinely shared as an encouragement to people to keep moving if possible, it is an example, albeit entirely unintended, of ableism, ageism, and fearmongering. And of course, it is not true. For an individual who has a condition that prevents them mobilizing their spine in any way close to the movement the teacher in the post was demonstrating, seeing such a post may be distressing at worst, and frustrating at best. It could even result in their thinking that aiming to be included in any movement modality is a waste of time.

I'm not only referring to people with serious disability. Someone with osteopenia, who knows it is unsafe to flex their spine to the degree shown in the video, even though they may be able to, might, at worst, ignore contraindications and sustain an injury, or at best be upset or fearful for their longevity.

I may seem to be overly judgmental here, and the likelihood is that not many people will have been upset by the post, but I use it as an example of the kind of advertising we see all the time in the yoga world that could benefit from a rethink, especially as we begin to teach people with menopausal bodies that may not be as able to bounce back from overstrain, or may be more likely to have limitations.

Of course, staying mobile is immensely important, but to suggest such simplistic formulae determine health or longevity is to create false boundaries, certainties, and fears. Nothing is that simple, and improvement of health outcomes and wellbeing are available to all, no matter their level of disability/ability, their weight, strength, age, or their flexibility.

A new approach to yoga for menopause?

Though honoring and valuing the tradition of yoga, I openly express that what I teach is not a deep yogic journey aimed at enlightenment. My intention is to use yoga as a tool to offer our organisms a more comfortable, pleasurable journey through the years, with a reasonable expectation as to what a body that has lived our life can do, and wants to do.

The core yogic principles I focus on are:

- Ahimsa/non-violence to self and student (safety over achievement)
- Satya/truth (no false claims)
- Koshas/layers of being (all layers welcome)
- Pranayama/breath work (selected)

- Dhyana/meditation (adjusted)
- Asana/physical practice (adapted)
- Svadhyaya/self-study (of our changing body, our reaction to those changes, and to societal pressures).

The following chapter constructs for you some possibilities of how yoga could be taught when the array of effects of the stages of menopause are taken into account, addressed, and sympathetically included.

This whole book contains what I bring to the yoga table: a reimagined offering that comprehensively and relevantly supports symptoms, perspectives, and the changing health needs of women in menopause. In each section, you will come to know how you may be able to speak about your work in ways that are in keeping with satya and ahimsa—in word, as well as in deed.

From reading about the relationship of stress to menopause, you will understand why the nervous system is at the heart of *Yoga for Menopause and Beyond*. So you will see that the tools that yoga offers in abundance to address nervous system regulation will be referred to again and again. And again.

Yoga for menopause is not all about avoiding stressors though! Because, in the right dosage, stress and cortisol are positive and necessary. We need to create "eustress" (positive stress) for our muscles, bones, brain, and heart. *Hormesis* is a word that I love to use to describe the phenomenon of eustress, whereby low doses of toxins (which in high doses would be fatal or damaging) induce a healing effect.

But the level of stress for the hormesis effect is different for each individual. So at the heart of yoga for menopause lie individualized recommendations. What stresses one woman negatively may be just the right amount of positive stress for another.

My conviction is that there is no absolute for the measurement of what is enough positive stress when it comes to our practice. One person may find cold-water immersion, for example, gives just the right amount of stress for a healing response, where for another this may be too much. This is why self-discernment is a key quality to encourage in all your students. Finding *her* hormesis may be the single most important focus you can encourage in a woman to help regulate her stress levels, and bolster her sense of self-agency, self-esteem, and her physical wellbeing.

We can also consider how we may be adding to a woman's stress because of the ways we teach, and the expectations we place on our students, albeit unwittingly. If we claim benefits that fail to materialize, encourage striving toward postures that may damage more vulnerable tissues, present esoteric practices that may feel unachievable or irrelevant to the average weekly student, or advertise ourselves as fitter, more youthful, healthy, and unflappably calm than our students, we may be adding to a woman's burden. Whether we intend it or not, the way we appear can make us seem like ideals to aspire to. Aims that involve trying to be more like someone else will almost always be frustrated anyway, but this is even more the case if how that someone else appears is skewed because of the "imperfections" she may be hiding.

So we do not add to the long list of "shoulds" in a woman's life, in our advertising, and in the tools we offer, we must aim to teach that which is achievable by most bodies, in most lives, during challenging times. Working one-to-one, we are also led by the individual, closely listening to her unique struggles and needs, and regularly checking with her how each tool makes her feel.

Being a yoga for menopause teacher of integrity is a broad undertaking, with implications not just for your time with your students, but also for how you attract them, and how you may affect the social pressures on women as they age. It is also a role with the most nourishing reward of any type of yoga I have ever taught. You will experience vulnerability, trust, encouragement, and gratitude from your students. They will feel more held by you than perhaps by any other, as they see you consciously caring for and valuing their experience. It is a privilege to hold women in this beautiful, difficult, devastating, empowering phase of the menopause transition, and the years beyond.

Please feel free to reach out to me, because you will need to support in holding these deserving women.

If you are interested in fascia, you will know what a tensegrity model is—an integrated biological form (bio-tensegrity) that upholds itself through a positive tension which enables the whole to function, rather than sections functioning independently of each other—figure 2.1. Health is like a biotensegrity: all you do to improve (or worsen!) one area of health will impact others.

This book is like an information-tensegrity. By which I mean that all parts of this book link to and support all other parts, and nothing that's suggested in one section is without impact in another. Thus, though I have tried to avoid too much repetition, some is inevitable, and I hope that this book will help you weave your own image of yoga for menopause. So, we begin to reimagine …

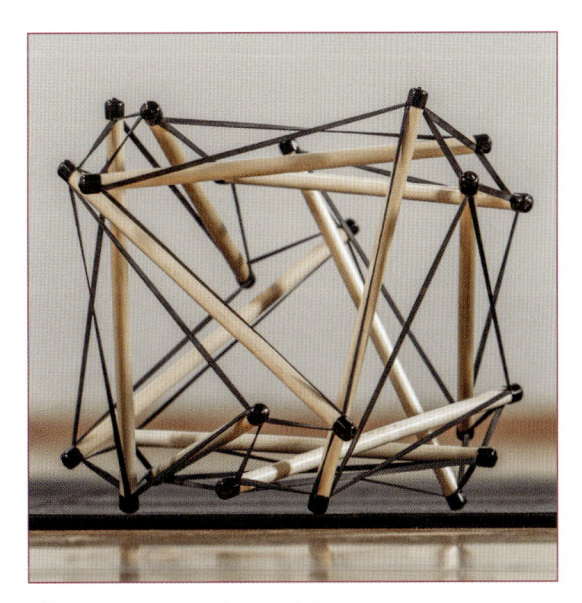

Figure 2.1 *Tensegrity model*

CHAPTER 3
A CLASS, REIMAGINED

If you look at the contents page, you will see that the order of this chapter broadly follows that of a normal yoga class (opening circle, warm-up, asana, rest, meditation, and pranayama). And why not?! Yoga classes are well structured already, and throughout them we use language to make clear our teachings. But in this chapter I will detail how each of these elements might be tweaked to avoid that which may harm, accentuate that which may help, and empower women to take yoga off the mat into achievable, repeatable interventions for the relief of symptoms and the support of relevant health goals.

A) AN OPENING CIRCLE, ENRICHED

Central to a yoga for menopause class is offering women the space to speak and delivering informed, compassionate information in response to what they share. Though these sharings can be long, and you will need to manage time sensitively, they are of immense value to women who have, possibly up until this moment in your care, been staying silent about their experience through shame or a sense that others have not wanted to hear them. Even without then offering information, this sharing with others who are truly interested and share the experience can be tremendously healing.

When you then add "aha moments" where women learn about why they are experiencing what they are experiencing, and suggest informed and achievable ways in which they might address these experiences and look after their health, you open up a world of perspective shifts and support which they may not have known were available.

The kind of advice you give may differ during the different phases.

The late reproductive stage and early perimenopause

During this phase, women often go for medical advice and leave with questions unanswered and fears unalleviated, because when menses is not more irregular than plus-or-minus seven days, perimenopause will not be confirmed. Learning from you about the LRS or build-up to perimenopause may help to normalize their experience and reduce fear. It's not joyous news to share, but it can be comforting to know they are not, as many report feeling, "going mad" or becoming unwell.

It may also be helpful to know about this phase because it signals that a woman is on the cusp of further change in her system—perimenopause itself. If she can accept what's going on, it can be an opportunity for her to begin to feel, rather than just intellectually know, that it's time to look after herself.

On a practical level, we can help with advice for liver health and gut health to help the body process and excrete possible surges of hormones. Supporting these and other health areas, as detailed in Chapter 5, may help her have a smoother perimenopause journey. You can help her see that this is more possible and less overwhelming than she might imagine, and that you are there to help.

It's also important to let women know that this is a time when getting some tests with their primary medical care practitioner is a good idea in order to rule out other possible issues.

Perimenopause

Offering empathetic, interested, and knowledgeable space for shared conversation or even one-to-one expression of her struggles may be the single most helpful thing anyone can do for a woman in the throes of her MT.

Many women report that, among other things:

- They hate themselves.
- No-one wants to listen.
- They feel they are going crazy.
- They think they are developing dementia.
- They feel alone.
- They are ashamed of their symptoms and changes.

The more they hear that their experience is shared, the less piercing these thoughts may become. All of the above list will be represented in any group gathered for perimenopause support. If you can create an atmosphere of trust where women are welcome to talk (or just listen), repeatedly and at length if your class or workshop allows, your class may become the only space where a woman feels that anyone is interested in what she is going through. Burdens will be released and self-value increased as she feels that you and the other women attending are at least interested and, more likely, fascinated by what she has to say.

Perimenopause is a time when some health challenges may be exacerbated, like issues with digestion or allergies, mental health challenges or hormonal difficulties like PMDD. It's not uncommon for women to be diagnosed with hypothyroidism or depression around this time, or to be low on iron. You have read that hypothyroidism has similar effects to perimenopause. Low iron can induce fatigue. Depression and chronic stress also share symptoms with the MT.

So, it's immensely important that you don't assume anything, or tell your student that what she is experiencing is definitely perimenopause.

Along with the tools and perspectives you will offer, and the unique and nurturing way you will hold your students, for your sake and theirs there must always be the disclaimer, 'This is not an alternative to medical care.' You would also be wise to find a moment to say, 'It's a time when a visit to your doctor to rule out any other possible causes and to get some routine blood tests is a very good idea.'

If we can begin to gently nudge women toward the need to monitor their health, while avoiding overloading them with scare stories at a time when symptoms can be challenging, then we are helping them to create a better outcome for the years post-menopause.

Postmenopause

Along with the information you share in the opening circle, primarily addressing the health of bones, brain, heart, and pelvic floor, you will be helping your students remain social, receive empathetic support, be heard and valued, and to maintain a positive outlook and a sense of purpose.

Ageism, ableism, and the cult of the slim, bendy body are contributing factors to the destabilizing nature of the perimenopause and later life. As you offer the tools that you feel happy to offer (after doing your research!), keep in mind that you want to create a resource that offers achievable practice that feels relevant, available, and adaptable as bodies continue to change. I have heard many women say that yoga begins to seem irrelevant or unwelcoming to them as the years go by. How lovely it would be if in the latter decades of life they could feel as at home in a weekly yoga class as their mothers may have done in a bridge session. Bridge is great, but the addition of research-based benefits of movement, meditation, and breath work, added to the perspective shifting, social and empathetic aspects, is a major plus for yoga.

B) A CONSTANT: LANGUAGE RECONSIDERED

> *I know this transformation is painful, but you're not falling apart, you're falling into something different, with a new capacity to be beautiful.*
>
> —William Hannan

In this section we look a little at the importance of how we communicate what we want women to know in class, and in advertising. In addition, suggestions on use of language have been peppered throughout this book and appear in subsequent sections. To offer some perspectives on the increased importance of words when caring for women in perimenopause and postmenopause, I offer you the following considerations.

In the work I am doing, countless times I have met women who are ashamed of what they are experiencing. It is my hope that those who are willing to speak out may begin to redress the balance so that those who are less vocal can journey through this time without the unnecessary additional baggage of shame.

Where has this shame come from? We have always been told that certain changes make us more valuable: getting fit, growing into our womanhood, losing weight, getting "better" at something, getting "control" of our body and emotions.

We have been told that certain changes make us less valuable: becoming softer in our body, "giving up" an activity, caring less about our appearance, spending more time alone, growing old, the cessation of fertility, expressing our anger or discontent.

In doing this work there are possibilities I hope for. Can we rewrite how we look at women in middle and old age? Can we embrace what used euphemistically to be called "The Change"? For change is all it is, and why should normal change be a source of derision, fear, shame?

I have been laughed at while hot-flashing, seen smirks on the faces of many as I described my brain-fog, listened to so many women saddened by their softening bodies, met ignorance about the duration of what can indeed be a lengthy, painful transformation. How is this the norm around a universal biological fact?

It's not the fault of one or two ignorant persons' lack of care, but a long-standing societal distaste for "women's issues" that has been the norm for hundreds of years. We are taught as teens that speaking aloud of our monthly bleeding is not okay, and we take that internalized shame with us through the years all the way to menopause.

Can we teachers help women to remember how beautiful they are, in all their manifestations, by working to strip away these years of conditioning? Can we see, and thereby help them see, the beauty of what they are, of what is emerging through change? The beauty of softness, of roundness, of emotion, of grey hair and soft flesh, of speaking truth, of getting to be alive still.

Perhaps we as teachers, male or female, can truly accept our bodies and the changes the years may bring, even to our yoga practice. Can yoga teachers take some responsibility for the perpetuation of the pressure to be infinitely capable and youthful? Can yoga teachers allow a softening of the physical fabulousness we demonstrate on our mats, and in our advertising also?

Can we as female or male teachers help ourselves and our students through the changes of life by being present, allowing ourselves to reach out for help, minding our health, and making our own decisions about what makes us valuable? Perhaps if we speak truth, society will be able to ease into understanding and acceptance.

Among the women in your classes you will encounter everything between those who know all about what to expect from their late 30s on, to those that believe that menopause is one chunk of time that will occur in their early 50s with the cessation of bleeding and a few hot flashes. Within that there will be:

- women who are hungry for education and truth, and those who want to avoid the details/avoid accepting it's happening in their body
- women who will be open to embracing the natural changes, and those who rail against them
- women who will be suffering huge and life-altering debilitation, and those for whom it is an easy enough journey
- women who want to talk about it, and those who don't
- women who will choose medical intervention, and those who avoid it or cannot take it
- and many variations in between.

So it's clear that how you speak of menopause is a hugely important consideration.

The more informed, compassionate, and open you can be with your own language, the better, while never assuming that your student is yet, or will ever be, ready to be as open as you are. In yoga teaching we lead by example. But just as in asana, this is not on the assumption that everyone will be the same or join us in our level of openness or lack of embarrassment.

Then there is the fearmongering. I'm going to step out of the middle of the road and be a little bit controversial here: it is inflated fear that drew too many women away from MHT 20 years ago, and now it is inflated fear that is being used to draw women toward it.

I'm not anti-MHT, I'm anti-fear. I use vaginal estrogen and I suggest to my clients that it might be wise to talk to their healthcare provider about the benefits of menopausal hormone therapy for them, particularly if they are very young, really struggling, or have a history of certain issues. Please read the section on medical interventions and you will see the balanced view.

This wild swing of the pendulum will, one day, calm. But for now, understandably, women's nervous systems are all jangled in the current atmosphere. This is, to my mind, creating discomfort and the lashing out that I witness in the menopause space.

I stick my neck out here again and say that I believe Big Pharma are always looking for new diagnoses for cohorts of the population so that they can give them reasons to be on medication for the rest of their lives. Using a term like "estrogen deficiency" sounds very much like a frightening diagnosis to me. There can be complications for some women because of the loss of estrogen, but menopause is not a disease.

"Deficiency" is a term that engenders fear and a sense of deterioration and of being less than we were. It implies that the only perfect state of female biochemistry is that of the reproductive years, and nothing before or after. Of course, on a species level, reproduction is our main function. But humans are more sophisticated than that, and to imply that post-reproductive females have outlived their function is to ignore the increasing lifespan of humans, even though it is so sought after. I believe that estrogen deficiency is a term that helps nobody and needs to be put aside.

If the narrative you read about menopause in the media is not upheld by specialists in endocrinology, the National Institute for Health and Care Excellence (NICE) guidelines, and statements from the North American and British Menopause Societies (NAMS and BMS respectively), I think it might be wise to ask who is creating that narrative, and how do they benefit from it.

The current generation of women in menopause are beginning to share and support each other like no other before. But, at the time of writing, there is also a danger of cementing a polarization that has emerged. Women are at odds as they find themselves judged for the choices they are making, or wanting to share and recommend the choices that have helped them, and sometimes judgmental of, or bewildered by, others for not choosing the same. I hope this is a momentary glitch in the dawning of a new era. But I am not certain, as the economics of pharmacology and monetized wellness culture may take hold.

As yoga teachers, we can be adept at holding space for many experiences and choices. But some of us can be judgmental of those who don't take a holistic approach. The way we hold space must be inclusive of all choices. We must also be ready to mitigate damage that may be unwittingly done by students in a sharing who express their judgements or opinions in ways that may not be as well-considered as someone with your skill.

Your teaching language

You may choose to offer your menopause supportive work overtly or obliquely. For instance, in a class of mixed ages and genders, you may choose to simply, quietly teach in a menopause-friendly and informed way, without ever making that explicit. If there are women in their late 30s in the class, rather than those in the middle of their peri- or post-menopause, in order to avoid an unwelcome barrage of information, you could help them prepare for this transition by recommendations such as:

> Now is the time for us all, but especially women, to be working on our bone density and muscle mass, because perimenopause and other factors mean our bodies get much less efficient at bone building.

You can see how you won't have put anyone under pressure, but will have piqued the interest of those who want to investigate further, and also popped something into the head of a woman who may remember it a few years down the line.

If you have a class of women from their mid-30s upward, it would be reasonable to assume that most women will be less informed than you are now. Some will be experiencing symptoms and know what's going on; some will be experiencing symptoms and not know why; some will have no symptoms. Being comfortable with honest and non-euphemistic language is key if you are interested in helping them come to a place of less fear and more acceptance. You may also, by your comfort in using language around menopause, empower them to feel able to advocate for themselves.

Consider sentences such as:

> When hormones begin their natural midlife shift, women may start to feel a lot more tired.

Or, if you yourself are a woman who has experience of menopause:

> In my research around yoga for menopause, I was so relieved to learn that my heavy bleeding was normal.

Or during shavasana:

> For a woman from her 40s on, rest after physical exertion becomes much more important. This is because, when reproductive hormone levels start to change, our body's recovery from physical and emotional stress takes longer.

Or during a meditation:

> In our 40s, life seems to present us with an overwhelming amount of things to juggle. This is true, but it can be worsened by the decline in certain hormones that usually give women their ability to calmly multitask. So, might we need to lighten our load?

These examples are clearly more targeted, but allow the women who are not ready to see where they're at, or who believe they are years away from menopause, to learn in a non-confrontational manner what may be ahead.

Clearly, if you have a group who are there specifically to address their needs during the stages of menopause, you can be more open. I would recommend that you limit your listing of the symptoms of menopause in order not to create undue worry, but do select a number of the less common or less well-known symptoms. It's a difficult balance, because your naming of an uncommon symptom could shine the light of understanding on something that has been a source of fear for one woman, but naming every single one may create fear of what may never occur for the majority.

It's my conviction that, in teaching yoga generally, and especially to ease the striving that can add to the depletion felt by women in this transition, we as teachers should offer rather than dictate. So phrases such as "if you like" or "if this feels good", or one I often use, "if this feels therapeutically interesting," give women permission to be responsive to their own needs and are an invitation to interoception.

Be conscious of your training and expertise. Unless you have other qualifications, you are a yoga teacher. Stay within your realm of expertise. It's okay to anecdotally report your own experience, but be willing and able to recommend other strategies, and to say, "I don't know the answer to that." It's important to be aware, for your own sake, that you can't fix everything, and to make that clear to your participants.

One of the greatest gifts yoga can bring is the power of self-discernment. Your greatest gift may be to simply clear the waters for a woman so that she can see what is going on, what she can reasonably handle herself, and what she may need help with. Further, this is a time when a woman could mistake medical issues for menopause symptoms, so it's important to put the diagnosis in a woman's own hands.

Think of asking the right questions rather than trying to provide all the answers.

All your participants will benefit from knowing that menopause is as individual as pregnancy. Just as one woman may have mild morning sickness and another be hospitalized with persistent vomiting for her whole pregnancy, one woman in menopause may have brain-fog, low mood and hot flashes and another may be dealing with depression, night sweats that necessitate changing her sheets, and joint inflammation that prevents her walking without pain. Some may be chatting about it freely to friends and have an understanding partner on their side; others with partners may even be too ashamed to tell them. No one's choices about how they support themselves should be judged, and no assumptions made.

A trauma perspective on language and teaching

You may wonder why there is a section on trauma in a book focusing on menopause, which is a natural transition. Let me explain.

The Cambridge English Dictionary describes (non-physical) trauma as, "Severe emotional shock and pain caused by an extremely upsetting experience." It can be something that makes us feel helpless, out of control, overwhelmed and unsafe in our body. Post-traumatic stress is when this reaction carries on for a prolonged time after the experience.

We know the Medusa myth: don't look her straight in the eyes or you'll turn to stone. So it is with trauma. Our organism says no to processing trauma all at once because it's too overwhelming. Instead it deals with it a little at a time. But if the mechanism of unwrapping and processing gets stuck, we can store it away in bits of our brain and in our physical body. Then we put control mechanisms in place to enable ourselves to keep it there so we can get on with life.

For a number of reasons, perimenopause can be a trigger for old traumas, which we have sidelined, to come to the fore. Our control mechanisms can be compromised by the challenges that the hormonal changes of perimenopause place on us physically, mentally, and emotionally.

Perimenopause may not be the time to face and deal with old trauma. So we need to protect our students from these triggers. If anyone becomes triggered, it's essential to seek help to manage the resurgence of trauma. Whether your client is on MHT or not, it's important to get professional help.

Most of us have experienced some kind of trauma. Some experts refer to "big-T Trauma" and "little-t trauma". Thankfully, most humans have not experienced big-T Trauma like war or childhood abuse. But little-t trauma doesn't even have to be direct trauma to you. Even hearing about or witnessing something like the sudden death of a family member or friend, or the serious illness of a loved one, is considered to have the potential to be experienced as trauma in your body. Many of us will have experienced physical trauma—an accident, serious illness, or injury. Even if we haven't experienced a dramatic trauma, many small repeated things may have made us feel unsafe enough to tighten up for self-protection.

We're more likely to hold trauma in our body if we resist our natural reaction. For example, if instead of making a stressor stop we override our instinctive reaction—like a child wanting to cry or shake when she's afraid, but instead being told to "get a grip"—we give confusing signals to our body that linger as tension in our tissues. One of the ways we deal with trauma is to become very head-oriented. In other words, we detach ourselves from the pain and uncomfortable emotions which manifest as sensations in our body.

Is menopause a trauma in itself?
When the body starts to experience perimenopause, women can be profoundly shocked at the realization that they are not as invincible as they thought. I know that when I was in my 20s and 30s, women over 50 were somehow "other;" they were not me in my future. In perimenopause, I began to recognize that I too had a body that would change and was becoming less of a reliable vehicle.

But more. When the buffers of estrogen and progesterone become thin, women can feel raw. And they are raw. Because what women are noticing is that they are not as in control of the outcome for their bodies as they may have mistakenly thought. Perimenopause can feel like someone has sent you a letter on headed notepaper and officially stamped, saying, "You are mortal." A woman may be awakening to the fact that death is there in all our futures. That sudden, embodied awareness could indeed be experienced as a trauma.

This sense of mortality often comes through her experience of fatigue, pain, anxiety, desolation, forgetfulness, and the feeling that she is "going mad." These experiences are potentially a trauma. Add to this some of the varied griefs that may be present in a woman, for instance if she still has a deep desire to conceive and give birth, and she can be forgiven for feeling profoundly challenged.

Remember what trauma can bring up: It can make us feel helpless, overwhelmed, and unsafe in our body, and when it lingers after the event, we feel out of control. Do those feelings remind you of anything? These are common feelings experienced by women in peri/menopause.

I believe perimenopause and menopause can be both a trigger of old trauma and a trauma in itself. Further, I am sad to say that there is growing evidence that women who have experienced adverse childhood experiences tend to have a more symptomatic menopause (Kapoor et al, 2020).

What makes dealing with trauma different for a perimenopausal woman than for a younger woman or a man?

During the reproductive years estrogen and progesterone help us to feel less pain, both physically and emotionally, and it's also a time when the human has "more important things to be getting on with." To make sure we get on with those things, we can be adept at hiding, denying, or pushing down feelings that are there, both for biological reasons and, of course, because society does not afford us the time nor the valuing of stopping and noticing, addressing and healing.

We all know that emotions have a physical effect on our body, and our muscles respond to difficult (and delightful) events to create a signature of muscular tone that is unique in each individual. We also know that just ... stopping ... or looking inward can be incredibly challenging. The picture of someone "keeping busy" to "get through" a period of grief, for instance, is one we all recognize.

So, in perimenopause our body is changing. One change is that it doesn't recover so readily after effort. It demands rest, and pause, and space. We can choose to listen to that demand and rest, or we can choose to try to "keep busy" and "push through." If we don't rest in perimenopause, we run a higher risk of burnout and fatigue. If we choose to respond to our body's changing needs, in that rest and slowing down, the body can start to relax. But when we relax the muscular tension our emotional life has created, and when we stop for perhaps the first time in our lives, uncomfortable feelings we have pushed down can begin to bubble up.

When we have the levels of estrogen and progesterone associated with the menstrual years, we have what you might consider the gift of their buffering us against the effects of physical, mental, and emotional stress. They are hormones which are necessary for the procreation of the species, but they don't just set us up physically to make another human. As you can understand after reading about the biochemistry, our sex hormones serve to make life much smoother than it might be without them.

In perimenopause a woman may not get the choice of whether or not to dive in and investigate, feel, and move through the trauma. Old trauma gets exposed at awkward moments, as the layers of blissful ignorance get peeled away. Sometimes perimenopause symptoms and midlife life-load mean women don't have the resources or the choice to say, "Not now, I will look into this trauma when I feel strong enough."

Like with Medusa, who can turn you to stone if you look at her directly, when we decide we want to heal from trauma, we need to enter her cave with a shield, and carefully look around the edges at first. Perimenopause can leave women feeling out of control and without a shield.

How you can help
It's essential to remember that if you're not trained in trauma therapy of some sort, you don't teach to try to release trauma. If trauma surfaces, your client needs trained help. But the lead author of another study about the effects of past trauma on perimenopause (Gibson et al, 2019) said, "Our findings suggest that routine assessment and *recognition of PTSD symptoms* and lifetime traumatic exposures when women are seen by healthcare providers *may enhance the effective management of menopausal symptoms*" (my italics).

I think recognizing that there is some struggle or vulnerability in our individual students, even if we don't know exactly what it is, is one of the abilities that many who are drawn to teach yoga possess. So you may already be helping. What we can do as teachers, as well as recognizing that the discomforts of trauma may be present, is to be conversant with trauma-sensitive teaching.

One of the most difficult things about trauma is the sense it creates of feeling out of control. To ensure your client knows they have some control, offer choices, especially around areas that are known to be potential triggers.

Someone suffering from anxiety may find it very difficult to be still, or to lie with their arms wide-open, or to welcome touch. Someone for whom old traumas are being revisited in this vulnerable time may find closing her eyes or focusing on her breath triggering.

The language must always be, *If it's okay for you to do so, close your eyes*, for example, and give other options, like, "If not, instead just drop your gaze" or even, "Feel free to look around and rest your gaze on something that interests you."

It may be helpful to say, "Focusing on the breath is not always comforting. If it's not comfortable for you, you could focus on …" Note that these suggestions don't predicate what the negative effect might be or why, so as not to trigger potential negative reactions.

I can't count the number of times, as a rookie teacher, I tried to persuade my students to take up shavasana exactly as I was taught it. If someone had their head turned to the side, or even lay on their side, bent their knees, had their hands on their belly, or had their eyes open, short of holding them to the floor in shavasana and gluing their eyes shut, I would do anything I could to persuade them into the "right" position. "Try it, it's *so* nice, and really relaxing," I would say reassuringly, probably randomly adding, "It's really good for you!" I didn't know then that shavasana is an immensely vulnerable position—for many, one of the most difficult moments in yoga—and the exact opposite of the stance we would take up under threat. Now, of course, I offer option after option, and the final suggestion to "take up whatever position would enable you to relax."

Orientation to our environment can help us feel safe. In particular, the brain trusts the eyes. So suggesting looking around a room and getting visually familiar with whatever areas of it are interesting to look at, before or during a class, or in shavasana, will help all your students feel safe. We may hope that our students can relax and inhabit themselves deeply and with attention. In perimenopause we will be hoping to reconnect them with a body they are coming to mistrust, or even hate. But that is a long, slow, scary journey for some.

Respect their trauma. Remind them, and yourself, that their need to stay protected is understandable and often wise.

Here are some techniques in trauma-sensitive guidance.

Give options for stopping the practice or modulating the intensity. For example:

- Open your eyes.
- Change posture.
- Take a few deep breaths.
- Take a break.

Give choices of where to anchor attention:

- Focus on what you're hearing.
- Focus on a simple physical thing (sensation in the hands, for example).
- Focus on the breath.
- Let go of focus on the breath.

Offer external anchors:

- Notice a tree outside.
- Notice a pattern on a wall.

You can assist your students by helping them to move their focus away from Medusa, by paying attention to what's right, or at least, what's okay, what's neutral, or what's possible …

C) A WARM-UP, HARD-WIRED FOR PLEASURE

Because of a tendency for synovial fluid to decrease in perimenopause and beyond, warm-ups which get it moving are more important than before. The practices in this section can be used for warming up or toward the end of a class, as a class in themselves, and can be lovely interspersed with postures in a yin or restorative class. Some may need to be kept back until a considerable degree of trust has been built, and your language may move from practical to imaginative to impassioned, as you and your students get comfortable with each other.

The kinds of movement you might teach in a warm-up, and those I offer you here, may be valuable also in caring for fascia that is changing (as detailed in the next section).

Somatic movement

Long before my training as a somatic education coach, I have been using movement practices that are adapted from what is known as Thomas Hanna's Somatics, and also from other traditions like the Alexander Technique and Feldenkrais, which I first benefitted from during my training as an actor in the 1990s.

Somatic simply means "of the body," so in effect, many movement practices are essentially somatic. However, I think it is possible to move the body with very little awareness, and somatics is very much about the mind–body connection, and the mental control of muscles. Personally I have found that a combination of 5Rhythms dance, somatics, and my somewhat outside-the-box yoga explorations, coupled with the changing needs and desires of my body in perimenopause, was the cocktail that helped me see that my yoga practice had not been nearly as embodied or conscious as I had thought.

I find that the kinds of simple, repetitive movement detailed below are an invaluable tool for the many people for whom movement does not involve the intimate collaboration of body, mind, and nervous system. I know I have been, like many students, someone who followed the line of, "Teacher tells me to do it, my brain makes my body do what teacher said, my body might get to have an opinion after I have pushed it into the required position!"

In my own practice and teaching, and particularly when teaching yoga for menopause, I use some formal exercises from my various trainings, some that I have created myself, and some that I have gathered from experiences over the years. I often then lead them in a way that allows them to morph into instinctual movement.

What follows are some of the exercises that I use.

Arm float

I first experienced this take on a familiar movement on a retreat with a teacher called Eleanor Dawson. This is a radical notion for most of our students. We are used to being instructed in every moment, and our body duly complies. Might it add to a woman's self-agency, self-esteem, and self-respect to notice that she has this kind of choice available to her?

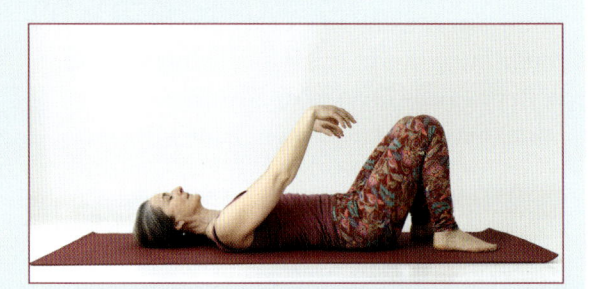

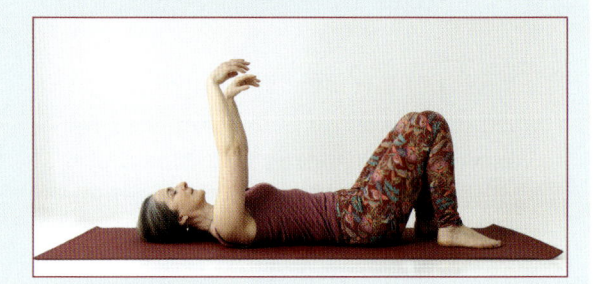

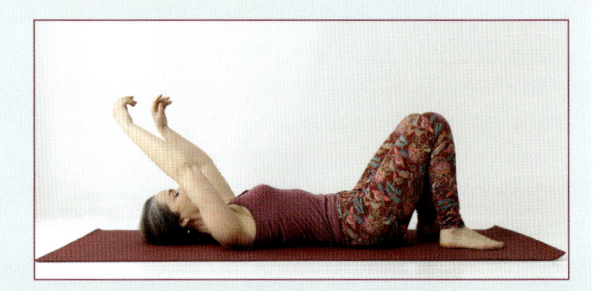

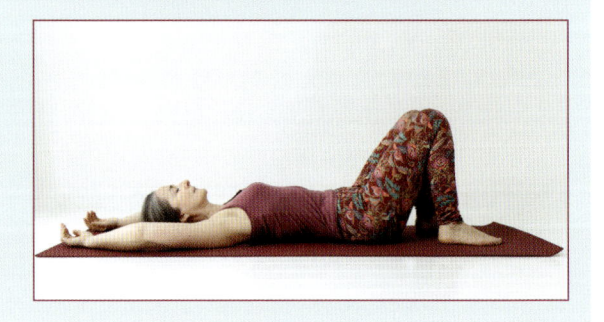

1) Lie semi-supine with arms by your sides. Pay close attention to your arms. Feel their weight.
2) Begin slowly to raise them up toward vertical on an inhale.
3) Lower them to the floor above your head on an exhale.
4) Inhaling, draw them back up to vertical and then, exhaling, bring them back down by your sides.
5) Notice the effect of gravity—when is it easy, when is it effortful. Notice the temperature of the air as you move through it. What else do you notice? Maintain the same attention and curiosity as you lower and raise them.
6) Repeat for a while.
7) Then let the arms journey all the way overhead, and back, in the same way. As many repetitions as you feel are appropriate.
8) Then, a whole new moment: With arms by your sides, taking as long as you like, give the arms permission to move or not … "Ask" the arms if they would like to move. See if they choose to do so. Notice when they want to stop. How far does the body desire to move, if at all?

Slow twist (or the Washrag in Hanna's Somatics)

I like to point out to students that in this practice the whole body is moving, to help them see the wide value of something so pleasurable (or at least restful and achievable, if they don't find it pleasurable).

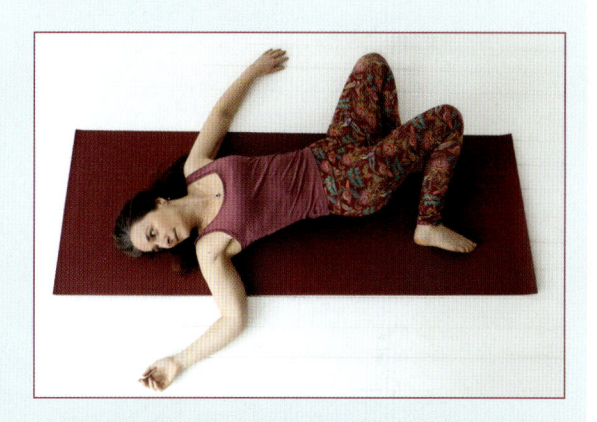

1) Lie semi-supine. Begin to let your knees move to one side, and then the other. Experiment with your breathing: perhaps inhale as the legs go toward the floor, and exhale as they rise. I usually suggest to students to exhale on the movement that's most effortful (because it is on the exhale that the core and pelvic floor muscles naturally engage).
2) After a while, add in a movement of your head in the opposite direction to the knees.
3) Once this is established, add in a movement of the hands, turning the palm of the hand that the head is rolling toward upward, the palm of the opposite hand down, moving if possible from the shoulder. Repeat multiple times.
4) Continue for two minutes or so. Rest, and tune in to the sensations in the whole body.

In the official Hanna's Somatics version, there is an intention to draw the knees slowly up and lower them slowly down by the movement of your spine and the muscularity of your abdominal muscles, creating rather effective core muscular demand and control. If you are using this movement for strength, which can be very empowering, you can add these possible cues I came up with: *Imagine you have a pulley system in your deep belly, and you are lowering the knees as you would a heavy drawbridge;* or *imagine a rope from your core to your knees with which you raise and lower them, as you would a lobster pot down into, and then up from the deep.*

Angel twist

Named the "angel twists" by one of my dearest students when I first introduced it to my classes back in about 2007, this is a lovely sequence for a class where your students are jangled, and you know that doing very little would be of value, but that they also like to feel moved in lots of directions. It can evoke memories of playing at being a ballerina as a kid. Or maybe that's just me! But I think doing this can help a woman to feel herself to be beautiful—at least, a beautiful mover.

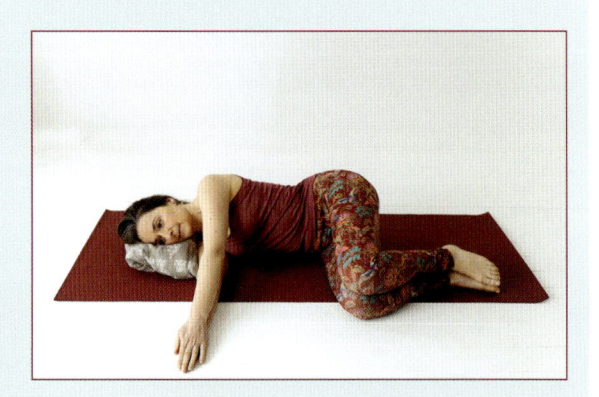

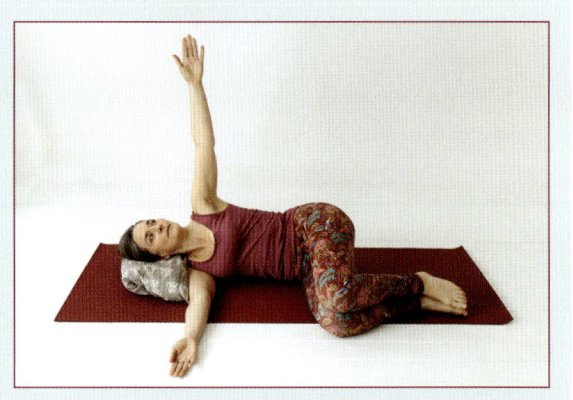

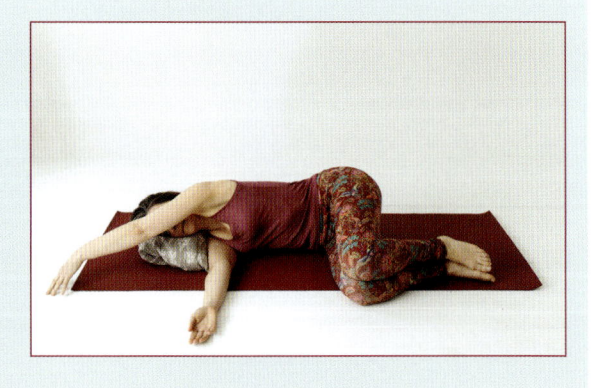

1) Lying on your right side, with a folded blanket or very low yoga block under your head, place your hands in front of your chest. Slide the left hand forward and take a few deep breaths into the left shoulder-blade area.
2) On an inhale, slide your left arm along the inside of your right arm and across your chest to touch the front of your shoulder. This may be the limit for some shoulders.
3) On an exhale, reverse the journey.
4) Do this 4 to 6 times. While doing this, I suggest that you notice the quality of the touch you are bestowing on yourself. What is the intention you have toward yourself in this touch? Can you imbue it with tender compassion?
5) Next you can allow that arm to fully unfurl behind you if the shoulder blade touches the floor first (without this detail, you may strain your shoulder because of the weight of your arm).
6) Repeat this a few times.
7) The next move can have the knees remain as they are, or the left leg can be extended on a very gentle diagonal behind you. As the left hand draws an arc on the floor above your head, the left knee draws up toward the navel. This movement may feel best on the

inhale, and return to center on the exhale. As with all breathing patterns with movement, allow your student the self-agency to do what she finds most helpful, pleasant, and/or safe.

As you continue, offer suggestions to stay aware of small sensations (once you have mastered the basic movement), and to notice what feels good about your experience. Always aim for pleasure over distance travelled, and enjoyment over looking for intensity or "stretch."

If there is spinal osteoporosis, the arm is unlikely to reach the floor because to keep the spine safe, the knees should be kept together.

8) Repeat as long as feels yummy! Rest in stillness afterward before repeating on the other side.

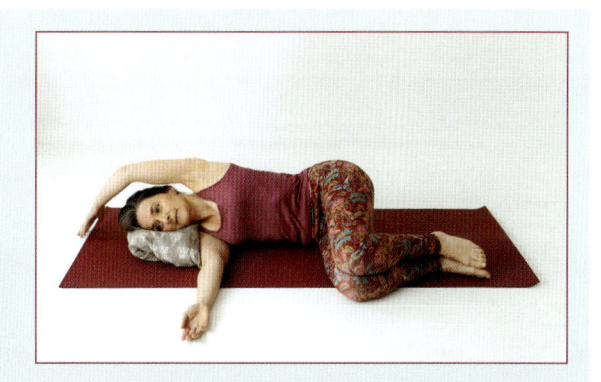

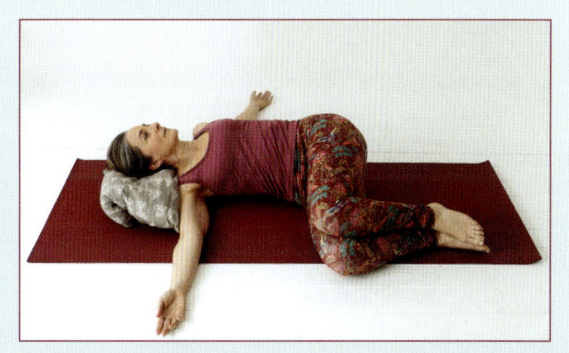

Yes/No

I need to withdraw … but I have to show up.

I may be giving this practice (its roots are in the Laban Institute of Movement) too much significance, but I find it a great metaphor for the struggle a woman has with feeling less inclined toward constant company, but an awareness that too much isolation is unhealthy in the medium and long term, and that there are still requests made of her that she may have to show up for.

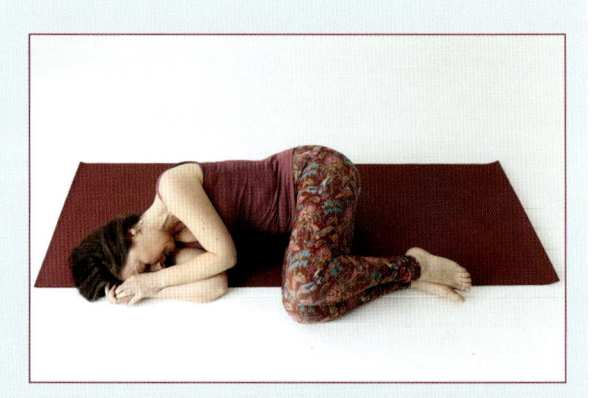

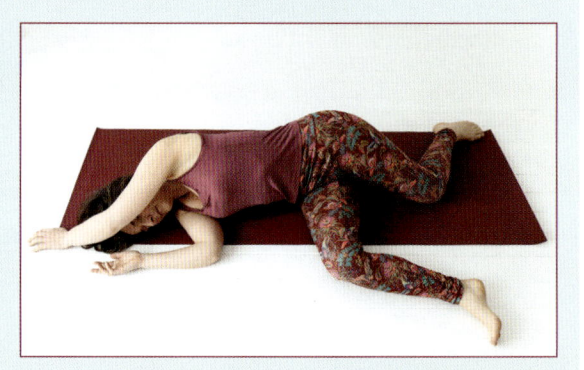

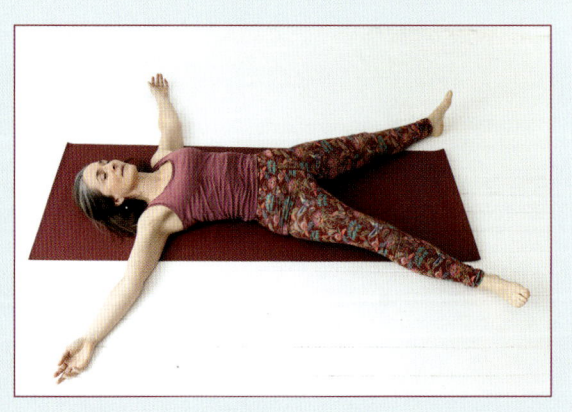

1) Lie on your side and curl up (less curl where osteoporosis is present).
2) Breathe and notice how it feels to be in this position. Here you might add some of the energetic awareness prompts below (in italics).
3) On an inhale, if it feels safe, roll onto your back and spread yourself like a starfish on the floor. Perhaps here you may speak about whether she is ready to stretch out, or needs to limit that movement (and other prompts from below in italics).
4) On the next exhale, roll onto the other side.
5) Repeat, moving from your side to your back to your other side.
6) You might want to move consistently with each inhale and exhale, or spend time in each shape.

Above are the basic movements, but there is so much more available, and your students may not complete all the shapes each time you teach this.

What can make this more than just shapes? Perhaps adding such prompts as:

> *As you lie on your side, how does it feel to be able to connect to your center, and show your back to the world?*

Is it helpful to go inward? Can you feel in your belly the nugget of strength that is always there, even in your vulnerable moments? Is it empowering to say no to the demands on you with your back to the world, and yes to connecting to the resources in your center?

As you roll to your back, does that feel good? If it doesn't feel good, allow yourself to curl back on your side. You can stay here for the entire time. Or you can play with moving toward that supine position by just extending the top two limbs toward the top and bottom of your mat, and then curling in again.

If it's nice to be on your back, does it feel possible to connect to the seed of joy that lies in your heart? It is always there, even in difficult times. Feel that seed of joy, sometimes more obscured, sometimes brighter. How does it feel to say yes to the world?

As you curl in, can you remember how it feels to unfurl?

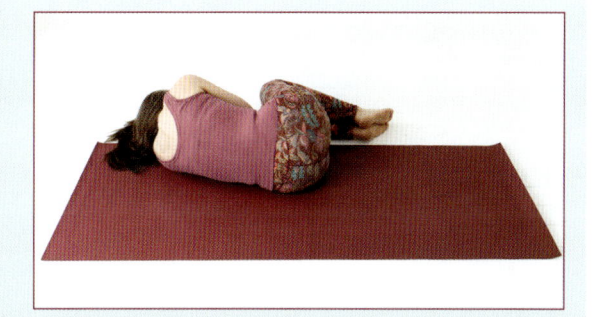

As you open out can you stay connected to your center?

Visualize yourself in a situation in life where you have to show up. Can you imagine being there, present, meeting your responsibilities, but, as if it's a photo of this moment in your back pocket, feel your connection to your center, and the permission to withdraw sometimes and say no.

7) Continue for a while, and then slowly wind the movement down until it stops, finishing in whatever position you feel inclined to stop in.

The sloth, or the upside-down leopard on a branch

I offer this practice to show the luxury of animal-like surrender. Getting the "dangling" energy of this is difficult for some, and sometimes doing only the arms or only the legs is more achievable.

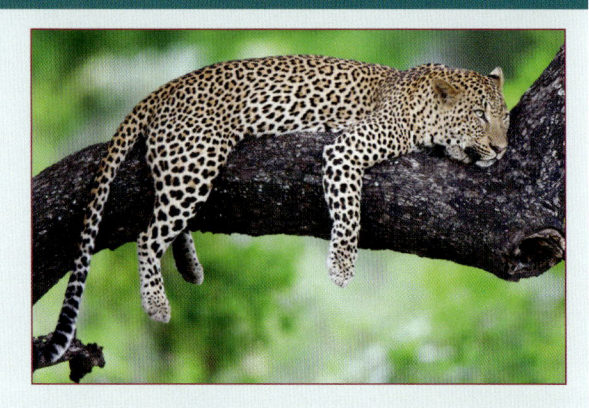

1) Lying on your back, float your legs up. I love to add the arms and melt my shoulder blades into the floor, but I notice that for some, the arms can't help reaching and stretching.

   You can offer this as it is, but I also like to use it as an introduction to feeling the layers of fascia:

2) Slowly begin to extend and flex at your wrists and ankles. You may be able to feel the layers of movement in your lower legs, and further up toward the hips and even lower back.

   How far can you feel the effects of this simple movement?

   The fascial layers move, not in the same direction but in opposing directions to each other. They slip-slide in reaction to one another, skin one way, adipose tissue another, deep fascia another, muscle another, periosteum (the skin of the bones) another.

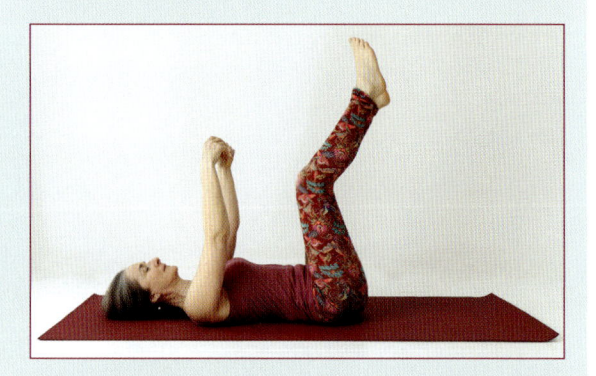

Feel them fluid. Feel how the layers love to move, and how movement aids movement.

You may have your own experience and language, or need to find something else to help them connect to movement, its subtlety and pleasure, if the qualities of fascia are not something you feel able to describe.

Banana pose

This in itself is from yin yoga, not somatics, but my students and I find it an achievable and really effective tool for the development of awareness of small sensations in many areas of the body.

1) In particular, I suggest you use the moment after the first side has been done for a few minutes. It is in the afterglow of the pose when sensations are particularly asymmetrical that you can help students learn and feel subtleties.
2) So, when they come back to center after the first side, suggest that they try to discover what feels different about each leg/hip/side of the trunk/shoulder, etc. Ask them to come up with words to describe those sensations. This kind of attention can then be suggested during their other physical practices, from restorative to robust.

These are delightful practices in themselves. They are also gateways into interoception and into self-led movement, as detailed below.

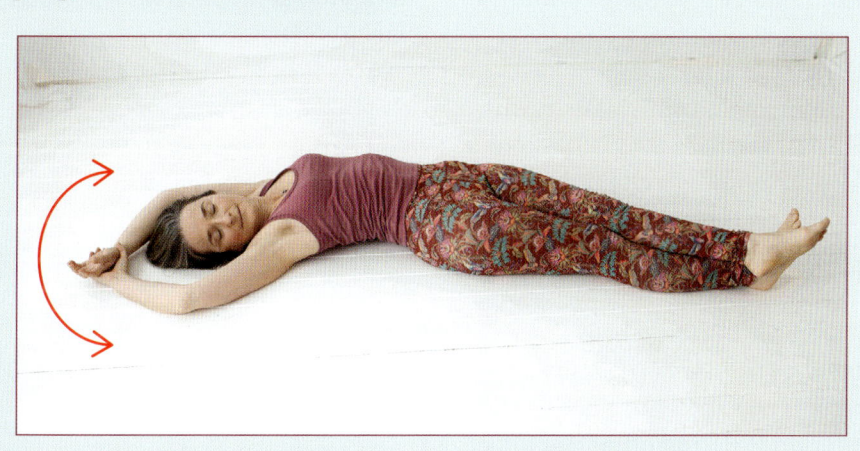

Pleasure and the feel-good hormones

In our warm-ups, when postural achievement is not yet on our radar, perhaps we can begin to help a woman reclaim the word pleasure, and the expectation of, and permission to feel, sensuality and pleasure.

Why is pleasure even more important in the stages of menopause than before?

Firstly, during menopause, especially during the unsteady, symptomatic time of perimenopause, a woman will often experience a loss of joy, and a reduced sense of taking pleasure in life, or of feeling pleasure in her body. This is something I am on a mission to address, helping women redefine their relationship with pleasure and what they think it is, but also noticing that it is still available. And it is not indulgent.

Secondly, many women find themselves intolerant of others, with less patience, perhaps a lessened maternal instinct, and an increased desire to be in their own company. This may be because of what you read in the biochemistry section, about the effects of menopause on hormones other than estrogen and progesterone, like oxytocin and serotonin. All of the "feel-good" hormones can be clinically or complementarily relevant in the alleviation of the symptoms and even health concerns of the stages of menopause. Pleasurable activities, rather than stressful ones, can induce them.

Endorphins primarily help one deal with stress and reduce feelings of pain. When they are in abundance we feel pleasure. Massage, exercise, and meditation, among other things, help with endorphin levels. Harte et al (1995) found that the effects of running and meditation on mood are similar, both producing endorphins and leading to positive feelings.

Serotonin stabilizes our mood, and promotes feelings of well-being and happiness. It impacts the entire body. It facilitates brain cells and other nervous system cells to communicate with each other, and aids:

- good sleep, by helping regulate circadian rhythms
- regulation of appetite
- learning and memory
- positive feelings and social behavior.

If levels are low you can experience, among other things:

- nausea and digestive issues
- irritability, anxiety, low mood
- sleep issues and fatigue
- cravings for sweets and carbohydrate-rich foods.

Serotonin production can be supported by meditation, exercise, bright light, massage (not necessarily professional), and mood induction (improving mood by focusing on positive things).

Dopamine is important in central nervous system functions such as movement, pleasure, attention, mood, and motivation. Positive levels of dopamine contribute to some things that are very pertinent to the stages of menopause:

- good digestion
- heart and kidney function
- memory and focus
- mood and emotions
- pain processing
- pancreatic function and insulin regulation
- sleep
- stress response.

Getting enough sleep, exercising, listening to music, meditating, and spending time in the sun can all boost dopamine levels.

Oxytocin, as well as supporting bonding, is an anti-inflammatory hormone; it can reduce blood pressure and cortisol, make us feel pain less acutely, and promote healing. Estrogen enhances the effect of oxytocin. You can see how relevant the less ready influence of this hormone might be to perimenopause experiences and later health concerns.

As teachers, we can encourage our students to aim for pleasure as much as possible, instead of stress-inducing improvement goals, and offer in our classes oxytocin-inducing stimuli like touch, warmth, social interaction, along with the receiving of empathy and support.

Outside our teaching we can point to the benefits of **hugs, empathetic company, listening to music you love (especially with someone you love), singing, eating, getting or giving a massage, sharing food with someone you love, having a cuddly pet, and orgasm**.

Perhaps more pertinent than any medicinal benefits from these hormones is the importance of helping your student remember that beauty, joy, and sensory delight are still available in this body of theirs. So we aim to increase joy and stay connected to the possibility of living with pleasure in our changing bodies. Suggest to your dear student to look for pleasure as often as possible by:

- Exercising in ways she actually enjoys
- Slowing down her coffee and cake: Advise taking time to really look at food, then smell it, then close her eyes and hold it in her mouth as long as she can, focusing on the subtleties of the taste before chewing really slowly
- Swinging her arms about and noticing the soft swoosh of the air on her hands
- Stroking her cheek with her favorite soft blanket
- When she notices something feeling yummy, stopping and tuning into it until it dissipates, rather than letting it stay in the background
- Meditating
- Pandiculating: Yawn-stretch like a cat every morning before she gets up, with the aim of feeling the pleasure of her body awakening, and then the deep surrender that comes at the end of that invigorating awakening of her musculature and nervous system
- When she feels like a yoga practice, suggest she try just lying down on the mat and moving in ways she wants to, rather than ways she thinks she ought to.

I hope you will be pointing out the benefits of pleasure at all stages in your teaching, but gentle as they can be, warm-ups are a great place to get started.

Encouraging truly embodied practice

During a warm-up, when students (and you as a teacher) are more used to play, and less concerned with the structure of postures, I would suggest introducing permission to improvise. This can induce a greater feeling of self-agency, and more likelihood of listening and responding to signals from the body saying "back-off" or "that feels good."

> When someone is struggling with post-traumatic stress disorder (PTSD) or post-traumatic stress (PTS), or is caught up in hating her body, interoception practices can be psychologically uncomfortable. Stroking one's own hand, tracing the fingers in particular, is a physical practice used in trauma support from trauma informed psychotherapy techniques, and this may be a less triggering place to start.
>
> I would also recommend stroking hands as a pleasure experience for all anyway. It can be a very gentle practice that ignites curiosity and tenderness.

Micro-movements

I believe these help my students feel pleasure, connect with their body, avoid injury, and avoid becoming disengaged from the experience of their organism as they move through yoga class or through menopause.

Tuning in to pleasure and avoiding pain may be more available if we offer tiny movements while in a pose, rather than feeling we have to freeze and hang on until we are allowed to stop.

Teaching micro-moving is difficult. Here are some techniques I have developed.

1) Beginning simply, on all-fours, I suggest making circles with the hips, which become larger and larger. Then let the movements become increasingly smaller. Keep making them smaller until the movement is almost invisible to an observer, so that you must tune in really attentively to detect any movement.
2) In an easeful version of pyramid/intense side-stretch pose (where the hands are perhaps on blocks or a chair to free up the joints), make lots of tiny shifts over the soles of the feet and notice how those shifts echo their way up the legs and into the hips. Next, make little or larger movements in the hips, like drawing figure eights or circling. Keep them subtle, with the aim of seeing what gives your hips greatest pleasure.
3) The simple balance challenges in the brain health section can also help us to notice micro-movements as we feel the minute shifts of the nerves and muscle fibers as they stop us falling.

Ask students to note these sensations, and the level of attention they bring to the body when balancing like that, and to bring that attention and those nuances when in another pose.

These can set the scene for women beginning to learn to respond to their body's suggestions; to let their body create its own movement.

Instinctual movement

Before leading improvised movement, protect yourself and your students by reminding them of contraindications for osteoporosis, or any other health concerns you know are present in the group.

Remember that once you have helped them to be more guided by their own body, you can add layers like:

> *Do you want to feel strong? Then perhaps you want to explore plank pose, or come up to a strong stance. Anything goes.*

Or:

> *Do you want to feel joy? How might you move to feel the openness and spaciousness of joy?*

Or:

> *Do you want to feel sensual? What would it be like to feel the touch of your hands on your face, or imagine the floor is a delicious fluffy surface to explore?*

What follows are some of the words and practices I use to help people begin to find the courage to improvise.

Yawn-stretch

1) This may be the easiest place to start. Lying down, I suggest that students imagine they have just woken up after a blissful sleep, and they have all the time in the world to indulge in a yawn-stretch.

As you encourage them to indulge in a prolonged yawn-stretch, remind them that pandiculation is something we see in the animal kingdom, and it has benefits to our nervous system and our tissues. Remind them also that they shouldn't look at each other, so they know no one is looking at them.

2) Lead as loosely as you can, but let them know you are there. Give small moments of silence that you can build on over weeks and months, interspersed with little suggestions like "How might you arch your back?" "How could you move your hips?" "How can you bring a twist to your spine?"

This is a great movement snack to suggest they take home with them and use every morning. Many women awake a bit achy, and doing this in bed before getting up can make a lovely difference.

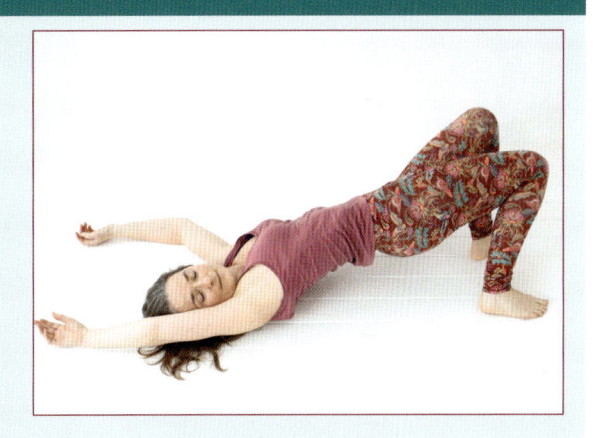

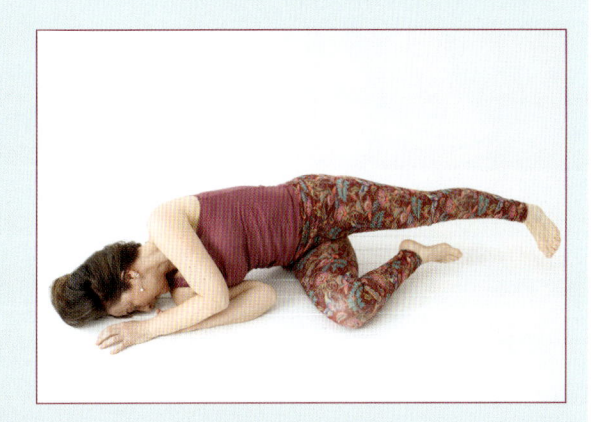

From all-fours

This could take some weeks to build up: Starting on all-fours can feel comforting because it's easier to focus inward and we can't see others. Again request that they don't watch each other.

1) Start with a simple guided practice of cat/cow, or hip circles. Say that at any point they can come back to this. Next you could suggest moving between two or three different movements in their own time, like cat/cow, or back to child's pose and forward to kneeling plank.

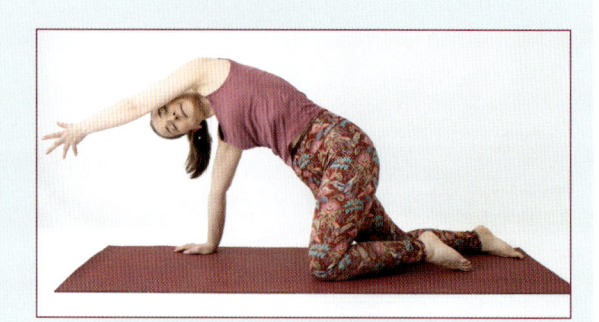

2) Then you could suggest seeing if they can create movements to fulfill flexing, extending, side-stretching and twisting. Then perhaps suggest their spine is a snake wriggling through long grass.

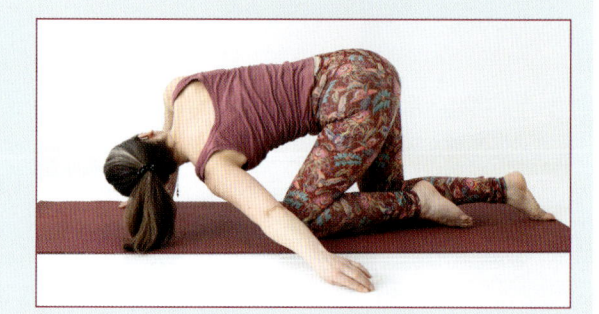

3) Finally, they may be able to move guided by their body. They can even find their way into downward dog, standing, lying, and absolutely anything they like! Suggest that they stay open to the body making the choice before the mind.

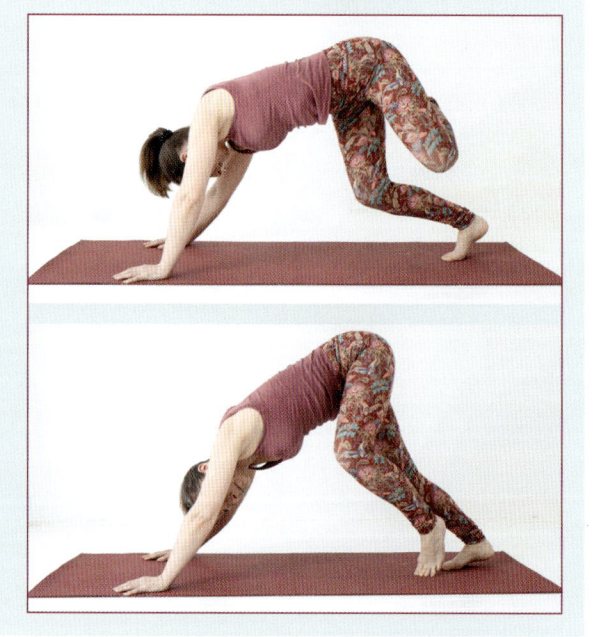

I recommend you make time in every class for self-led movement, whether that's for 30 seconds during a warm-up, a few minutes during a flow of asana, or for a time just before shavasana when you could suggest they move freely to enjoy some desire for movement that hasn't been satisfied in the class.

> *Offer a few ideas: Does your body want a twist perhaps? Maybe you'd love a last cobra? Maybe you're longing for a handstand! And encourage: What happens if you let your body move before your brain decides? Can you follow your body before your logic?*

Most of the practices in this warm-up section can be done without, or used as part of a warm-up, and they don't take up too much time. This makes them an easy, pleasant go-to for a daily self-practice for a busy multi-tasking woman.

D) ASANA, RESPONSIVE TO CHANGE

Even outside of menopause, we know that yoga asana can injure (Lee et al, 2019; Swain & McGwin, 2016), just as any exercise can. Unfortunately we hear of some yogis of all ages suffering with issues that would normally beset an older population, such as bony spurs, labral tears, need for hip-replacements (Parkinson, 2019) and sacroiliac joint (SIJ) dysfunction. These are issues that can occur from instability and/or excessive mobility (rather than strength) around the spine, hip, and SIJ respectively. Avoiding injury, and the cascade of negative effects it can engender, is always wise, but more so in peri- and post-menopause.

Whether they have incurred injury or not, for *some* women, continuing their asana practice in the same way as they have practiced during their menstrual years may be sustainable. For most—at least, for the vast majority of students and teachers with whom I have worked—it is not.

Some practitioners find that, instinctively, their practice changes if they listen to the changing reactions of their body, not just to avoid injury but also to honor changing energy levels and to bring them pleasure. Others continue, ignoring subtle signals, until, unfortunately, they get injured or disheartened.

A teacher can indicate that there are structural and energetic reasons for adjusting an asana practice, and at the same time make clear that such adjustments do not preclude much of what their students love about asana. We can still make fun shapes, play with arm balances, find creative ways to go upside-down, challenge our strength, and maintain our mobility. If this is made clear, then rather than feeling like a loss, it may feel more like what it is: intelligent, adaptive change, full of potential. Thus, the acceptance of these adjustments could be of broader benefit, not just by the avoidance of depletion or injury, but also by a greater willingness to adapt to, rather than fight the life- and body-wide changes arising.

So what are the physical reasons for considering change in an asana practice? Among many things still being researched, from perimenopause onward, there is reduction in cartilage and synovial fluid, changes to muscle and fascia and to the quantity and behavior of collagen (the building block of all our tissues). This means that exercise, including asana, can be differently impactful, and women can be more prone to injury, poor repair and/or prolonged repair time (Enns & Tiidus, 2010), fibrosis, and inflammation.

> *ECM [extracellular matrix] stiffening, induced by increased collagen deposition, especially collagen-I and cross-linking, disrupts normal tissue morphogenesis [tissue shape]. In parallel, during menopause collagen-III and fibrillin [responsible for elastic fibers in collagen] contents decrease in a statistically significant way, reducing the scaffolding which assists the alignment and*

> *cross-linking of elastin molecules, and consequently **decreasing the elastic properties of fascial tissue.*** (Fede et al, 2019; my bold)

To date, areas of the body that studies have shown to be more vulnerable to injury in peri- and post-menopause are around the shoulder, the knee, the pelvic floor, and the Achilles tendon. There is also a small amount of research into a greater tendency toward pain around the greater trochanter. I certainly notice a considerable proportion of the women I work with experiencing bi-lateral hip pain.

Systemic inflammation is generally higher in perimenopause, leading to greater likelihood of a dysregulated inflammation response to injury. Indeed the risks for agitation/inflammation of all tissues may be higher (Abildgaard et al, 2020). Systemic inflammation is when the body is on high alert to create a defensive response (inflammation) where it may not be necessary. It may manifest, for example, as all-over pain, fatigue, digestive issues, frequent illness, and weight gain.

Increased inflammation may be the main culprit in joint pain, and why a woman would be advised not to simply try to target individual areas of the body, but to address other factors like diet and stress that can increase inflammation. You may also see why our offering practices to "open the hips" or increase flexibility in the shoulders, for instance (as a reaction to a student complaining of stiffness or aches in these joints), may now be too simplistic a solution.

Cartilage decreases, making us more prone to cartilage tears and arthritic pain if we take the joints to the end of their range of motion (Roman-Blass et al, 2009; Wluka et al, 2003).

If osteoporosis has been diagnosed, there are additional risks for injury. We will go into this further in the section on bone health.

How do we know if we are going too far for the joints? How do we cue to avoid impingement and damage to cartilage? Stop if it hurts? Possibly. Though many of us have a strange relationship with pain, especially if we grew up with the mantra "no pain, no gain".

But what if we do understand and listen to our pain signals and act to stay safe? Will that ensure we don't put too much pressure on our joints? Not necessarily, because cartilage has no nerve endings. Let me say that again: cartilage has no nerve endings. What does that mean? It means we don't sense excess pressure when the cartilage is robust. But we do, and painfully, *after* cartilage is torn or has deteriorated. Then … it's a long road to recovery, and rebuilding may not be possible in the latter half of life.

So, we cue our students to look for other sensations: uneven levels of pressure in either hip, shoulder or knee; a sense of isolated stuck-ness (I feel impingement like a nut stuck in my hip); a sense of weakness or collapse in joints, rather than an ability to hold the body up (see pigeon pose, p. 82); difficulty getting out of a position; achiness after postures; isolated areas of intensity.

In general, I would aim for engaging in postures with strength and control, rather than hanging out "surrendered" and/or "dropping" into a shape (unless it is fully supported, as in restorative) and aim more for widespread rather than small areas of intensity/sensation when inhabiting any posture.

Exercise in general

For a woman who is already experiencing poor sleep, or is stressed, fatigued, has reduced lung function and/or is experiencing raised inflammation responses, endurance or intensive exercise can contribute negatively to her struggles, symptoms, and health.

An appropriate movement practice is, as ever, important for wellbeing on physical, mental, and emotional levels. Women may benefit if exercise is adjusted to address the increased risk of sarcopenia (loss of muscle mass), bone density loss, joint stiffness and pain, cartilage reduction, fascia stiffening, and depression from reduced serotonin levels.

The loss of self-esteem that can accompany the experience of the changes in physical and mental wellness would lead us to recommend an exercise protocol that is *achievable*, stress free, and enjoyable. In fact, statistics indicate that men exercise more because they *want* to, and women because they feel they *should*, mostly for weight and shape management. An interesting study into the effects of exercise among men and women, taking into account the reasons for exercising, found that:

> *exercise alone may not be beneficial under all circumstances for women ... for women ... there was a trend toward significance in the model assessing the combined effect of exercise habits and motives on quality of life. Thus, there may be some additional benefit to encouraging women to exercise for reasons other than to change body shape through toning the body or to appear more attractive.* (Craft et al, 2016)

This points to the value of offering exercise that is not about achievement, but more about how good it can feel, especially when we do so without pushing.

As with nutrition, so with movement: the human body and mind respond well to *variety*. So it behoves us as teachers not to promise that yoga can address all of a woman's movement needs. It is also worthwhile to "change it up" in class, so women are not repeating the same asana over and over every time they practice. Your students may also benefit from a gender- and age-specific weights program and some form of cardiovascular exercise.

Oxygenation is important for stimulating the mitochondria in our muscles to give us energy. So, considering possible lung function changes, increasing oxygenation through deep breathing practices and enjoying sustainable aerobic activities, perhaps with moments of gently increased effort—walking uphill, or walking faster for a minute or two every now and then—may also assist with energy levels and enliven a slower metabolism.

Though cardio, in the form of moderate jogging, walking, hiking, and/or swimming, remains beneficial for physical and mental health, we see the importance of exercising less intensively, and focusing more on functional mobility and muscle strength.

If that is not an acceptable option for an individual because, for example, endurance runs are her go-to for mental health, we can emphasize the importance of bringing stress levels down again as soon as possible after exercise. For instance, taking a stroll after a run, sitting looking at the view at the highest point of a hike, or doing gentle yoga or breathing after the gym.

Next we will address how in our teaching we can reduce physical triggers to stress and/or injury.

Functional yoga in the stages of menopause

Taking all this into consideration, it is my conviction that functional yoga (with a small f, because what follows is *my* version of a growing trend) is more beneficial than some more one-size-fits-all physically adventurous styles as a support for ongoing strength, mobility, and comfort in life, especially for times when our body is challenged.

The dictionary definition of the word functional (as supplied by Oxford Languages to Google) is "of or having a special activity, purpose, or task" or "designed to be practical and useful, rather than attractive". I am most definitely a fan of function over aesthetics in yoga, and for it to have a purpose outside of the postures, and even outside of the end goal of enlightenment. I admit to being, perhaps, more of a user of yoga than a yogi, just like most weekly students who are there to enhance the comfort and functioning of body, heart and soul over their lifespan, i.e., functional yoga.

Average-onset menopause segues into the decades when our bodies may become less reliable and less capable of the functions required to live independently. Physical yoga practices for postmenopause should, to my mind, be aimed at maintaining the ability to reach to the top shelf in the kitchen or put our socks on.

When considering functional over aesthetic, I tend to ask myself the question, "Would I do this in life?" My approach could be called Paleo-Yoga! Is there anything about the postures I'm aiming for on my mat that a Paleolithic human who knew nothing about the "need" to stretch or exercise would actually do?

Let's take wide-leg forward fold, for example. If I was sitting on the floor and I needed my (Paleolithic) spectacles (eye-glasses)—in order to read my Paleolithic text book!—I would lean over to get them.

But if I was sitting with my legs wide would I reach forward with straight legs, leading with my chest and thinking that the pull in my inner thighs was "good for me?"

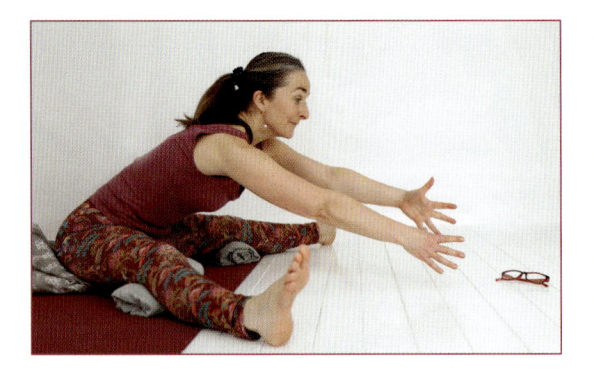

Or would I just bend a knee, and get my bottom off the floor a bit to reach them quite naturally and without intensity?

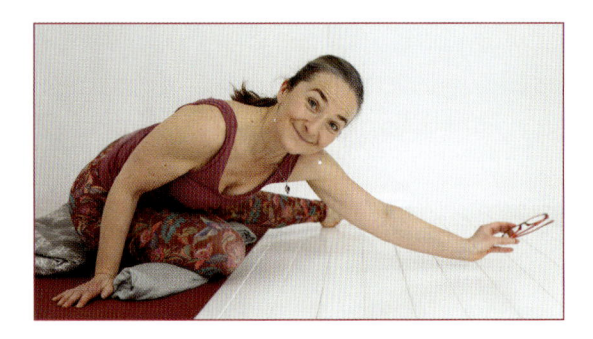

What would happen to your practice and teaching if you asked yourself, what's the point of this posture? And how might your considerations better include and support someone with the concerns of peri- and post-menopause?

Stretching

Essentially, the job of a muscle is to contract to enable movement. Its job is not to stretch. In fact, according to my study with world-renowned clinical anatomist John Sharkey, he (and many, many other experts) would say that muscles simply *don't* stretch. They contract concentrically (toward the center, as in a biceps curl where the biceps looks shorter and more rounded), they contract eccentrically (away from the center in a rearrangement of muscle fibers that creates a lengthening of the muscle's appearance, as in a bicep curl where the muscle goes longer and flatter when we slowly lower the weight), and isometrically (where there is contraction without lengthening or shortening, as when you push against a wall).

Passive stretching is when we use gravity, a strap or a hand, or are manipulated by a teacher, to get into a position that could not be achieved by unaided muscular effort. It is a hotly debated topic, but there is some evidence to suggest that static, passive stretching at the end of range of motion—the kind you might see in wide-legged forward fold where a student is pulling their toes in an effort to bring the front of the trunk toward the floor—is not optimal for our muscles (Smith, 1993).

Sharkey and others say that the reaction of muscular tissue to any request to "stretch" is to contract. In fact, I have heard some movement professionals theorizing that the pulling intensity we feel (and call stretch) in a pose is actually the sensation of those muscles contracting. Trying to "go further" may induce a weakening effect because we are asking our muscles to go places they aren't inclined to go, overriding their natural function, while they try to contract—which, theories suggest, makes them "give up". This weakening is known as muscular inhibition, where muscles become, for a short time, uncontractible. This may happen in yoga more often than we would hope and, in this moment of inhibition, injury can occur to other muscles which are having to overwork to make up the deficit.

When we override that natural impulse to contract by using force, such as being pushed by a teacher or pulling on a strap, that can also feel unsafe and we may lose the trust of our nervous system, which is trying to protect us from injury. A worried nervous system puts the brakes on; reduced mobility is an effect of the stress response. So we may do the opposite of what we want to do (ease tension, increase mobility and strength, and reduce pain) because the muscle becomes defensively tense to protect joints or soft tissue.

As I say, although this makes absolute sense to me, it is a hotly debated topic, but you can decide for yourself if you read Brad Appleton's in-depth online study (Appleton, 1996). You may also be interested in Brooke Thomas's podcast discussion on this subject with John Sharkey (Thomas, 2016).

Even if you don't agree about the risks of stretching in the general population, there is definitely a cohort for whom stretching is very risky. Hypermobility syndrome, which causes laxity of the support structures of joints, can become more problematic in perimenopause (Perry, 2019). Very little research has been done on exactly why that it is. Whatever the connection, this would be a time to avoid prioritizing ever-increasing range of motion in yoga class, given that a considerable number of yoga lovers are hypermobile.

Going further into a yoga-type stretch is perhaps an interesting thing to do if you want to achieve a complex asana or you are a gymnast, but may not be necessary or beneficial for a comfortable life in the long term. Gymnasts and ballet dancers know that their careers are often short, and what they do can result in injuries and chronic physical problems.

A very interesting study (Wyon et al, 2013) showed that of three cohorts of dancers, a group who stretched to 30% of their possible exertion (i.e., avoiding pushing or pulling themselves into stretches) and another group who engaged in strength training (i.e., using muscle strength) developed improvements in both passive and active range of motion, while a third cohort, who stretched to 80%, improved only in passive range of motion, not in active.

This is an enormously important finding because it is *active* range of motion (i.e., mobility without the aid of gravity or external forces), not passive, that we need to maintain to live life functionally. We don't need or use passive stretches to perform *anything* we need to do in daily life. We *do* need active range of motion to do anything from climbing a stairs to picking up our keys from the floor, to getting food from a cupboard. *Everything*.

So, in yoga for menopause I encourage avoidance of stretching as an aim in itself, focusing more on mobilization and on maximizing strength and support. Now we will look at how to practically focus our asana teaching toward these goals.

One way is to consider how to increase muscular effort in asana. There are three types of muscular contraction, as listed above. There is value in adding repeated movement in your teaching to encourage concentric and eccentric contraction. These contractions are present even in somatic movements, and you can add more muscular activation by encouraging slowness and smoothness of movement, and imagining resistance, or even adding resistance, as you will see in Chapter 4 a).

There are already lots of opportunities in yoga for increasing isometric contraction (IC) because it's naturally there in many poses, though often at a less intense level than might be optimal for our cohort. Isometric contraction occurs when we push against an immovable object. Isometric stretching involves that pushing, but occurs when the limb is at an angle that constitutes a stretch (for instance, elevating a leg onto a table and pressing down with the heel). Activating muscular contraction in a stretch may reduce the likelihood of "going too far" and this greater muscular activation may even offer better results (Wyon et al, 2013).

In case I haven't yet convinced you of its worth because of the strength it adds, isometric exercise has also been seen to be the most valuable type of exercise for reducing blood pressure, so important when aiming to support the health concerns of postmenopause. We can easily use IC to add muscular demand in postures where we linger for a while, like in the standing poses.

Below, I break down a few familiar postures, and discuss how common ways of teaching them may be unhelpful to women in peri- and post-menopause (and even, I believe, to any practitioner), and how we might improve their value.

Triangle

Not everyone's Triangle will look as crumpled as this, but I would guess that you see this kind of shape regularly in your classes.

1) Aiming for the floor, we may create deep compression at the front hip (usually, at this range, including pressure on thinning cartilage), a strong pull to the hamstrings with the SIJ out of natural alignment, often a side-arched spine and a neck straining to see the elevated hand.

   Coming this far toward the floor means there is flexion, side stretch, and twist in the spine, making this contraindicated for osteoporosis.

   There are many areas which could be struggling despite plenty of value being available from this pose at more natural ranges of motion.

   Look at these adapted versions.

2) Here we come into the posture at a more reasonable range of motion for our unique hip socket, femoral head and neck relationship. This is done by tuning in very specifically to the motion of the pelvis in relation to the femur, and ensuring that we stop the moment that hip movement is felt to reach its natural end point. Think Paleo: Stop when you reach a movement in the hip where in real life you would likely rearrange yourself (perhaps pivot the back foot, bend the front knee, or kneel down) to reach the floor.

In this pose we often see a hyper-extended knee (I'm not capable of that!), which can destabilize one of the joints that is most prone to injury in postmenopause.

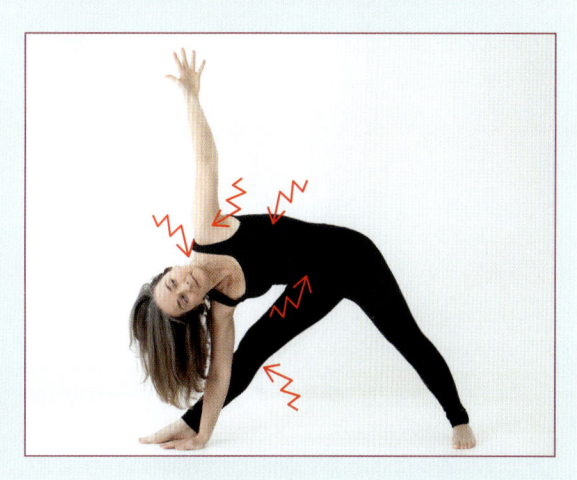

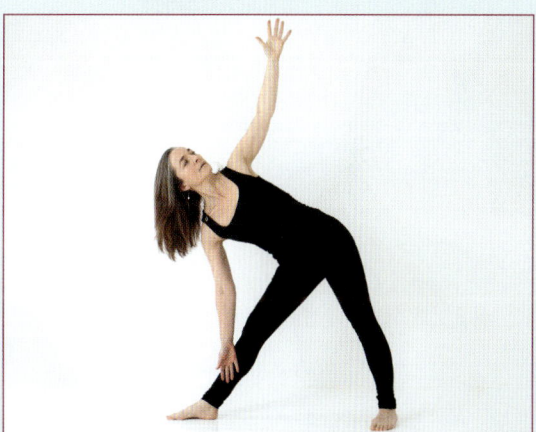

Then we check for the sensation of impingement or pressure in the front hip, and check for locking or hyperextension of the knees (in fact, a micro-bend in the knee will not only reduce the risk of hamstring tearing or over-stretching, it will also engage the support structures of the knee itself).

If no hyperextension or impingement seems present, we can assume safety, and then we can focus on the tone of the legs. Here, and in warrior II and in half-moon later, I would use cueing like: *Allow the back hip to roll forward a little*, which values the safety of the SIJs over the aesthetics of hips in line with the side of the mat.

3) A block for the hand is not always necessary, but may help reduce the striving to reach the floor. If there is shoulder or neck pain, the arm and head positions in the version with the blocks are usually achievable.

To help a student understand the principle of isometric stretching, suggest she draw her attention to her legs and ask herself: Do they feel tired or at ease, effortful or relaxed? Then suggest she makes efforts to push the floor away with her feet, and tune in again to the feeling in the legs. You might also suggest that she draws her muscles into the bones, particularly those of her thighs (most accessible in terms of feeling), like air being suctioned out of one of those vacuum storage bags!

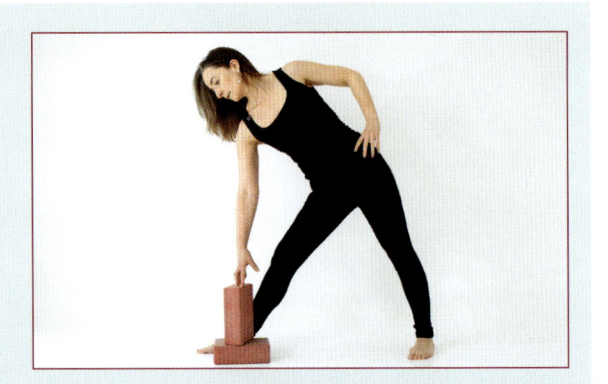

You may have heard cues, in warrior I for instance, like *Imagine you are trying to tear the mat apart with your feet*, or *Imagine you are trying to scrunch the mat up with your feet, pulling them toward each other*. This is cueing isometric contraction.

Search for your own images to help your student find activation in the muscles. You can suggest that if she feels she is making more effort than before, and that she would become tired if she continued, she is on the right track.

Warrior II and III

In this first version, I placed my feet so wide for the photo that I felt unstable, yet they don't look nearly as wide as is commonly seen in warrior II.

1) I pushed down through my hips (poor pelvic floor, poor hips!) and reached passionately through my arms (poor neck, poor shoulders!). It felt awful. Just bringing the feet a little closer, pressing down through the feet to rise up, and softening my arm reach soothed every bit of anatomy that before had felt "poor me!".

It can still be strong though. Even before arriving at the expression of the pose for each individual, the movement in and out of these poses can be adapted to maximize muscular use. Suggest to your student that as she goes to bend the knee she aims to imagine resistance to the movement.

> *Phrases such as Imagine resistance as you bend the knee may suffice to someone who is in tune with the nuances of movement, or images like Imagine there is a heavy box in front of your knee that you have to push along the floor may be better for someone newer to physical practices.*

Find your own ways, but ask her to imagine that the resistance is continuing throughout the time she is in the pose, while continuously encouraging the pushing of the floor away with both feet.

Note: For all sorts of reasons, but not least to help your student to a sense of self-esteem, of honoring her body, and coming to a capacity for self-discernment.

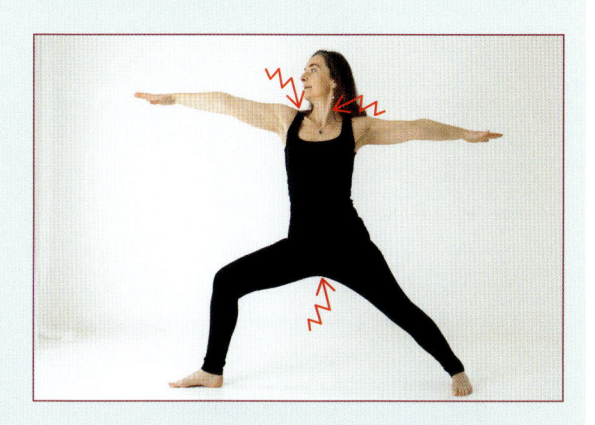

2) I assume that you will be constantly offering her ways of adapting all postures to ease any niggles, and modeling that in your own demonstrations, as in the adaptation of warrior III in the second image, rather than modeling the adapted versions for a bit and then settling in the "full" version yourself, as if this is the most valuable one that everyone should aspire to.

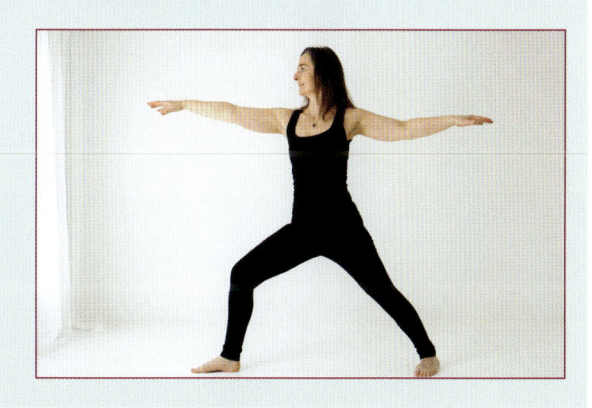

3) In both versions here, the standing knee is micro-bent, adding to muscular engagement, and the pelvis is lifting up off the femur, to reduce pressure on the hip joint.

I often teach this with hands on the hips or softly dangling (try it—it can release intensity from the shoulders and adds a yin feel to a yang effort). Remember to assure your student that even if she is performing the more upright version she is still gaining great benefits. If she is challenged, but not out of control, the positive stress her muscular and balance systems are getting is enough for her hormesis.

As you practice the new intensity of isometric contraction through the legs in all standing postures, you may also notice less of a tendency to collapse into the joints in these and other asana. This will aid in maintaining safety through the engagement of the joint support structures. Thus, you will reduce the risk of bone-on-cartilage pressure in regions already lacking in the fluids and cushioning required to protect the joints from wear and tear, and subsequent pain.

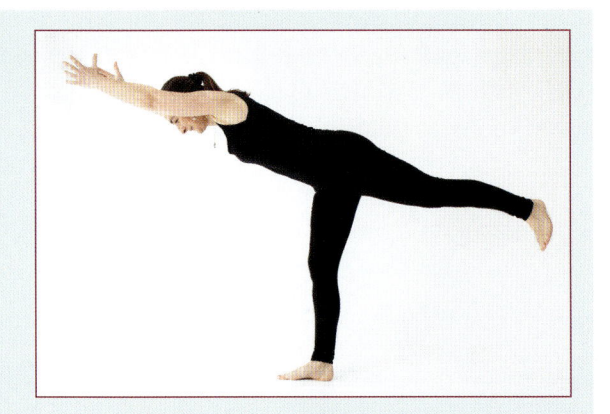

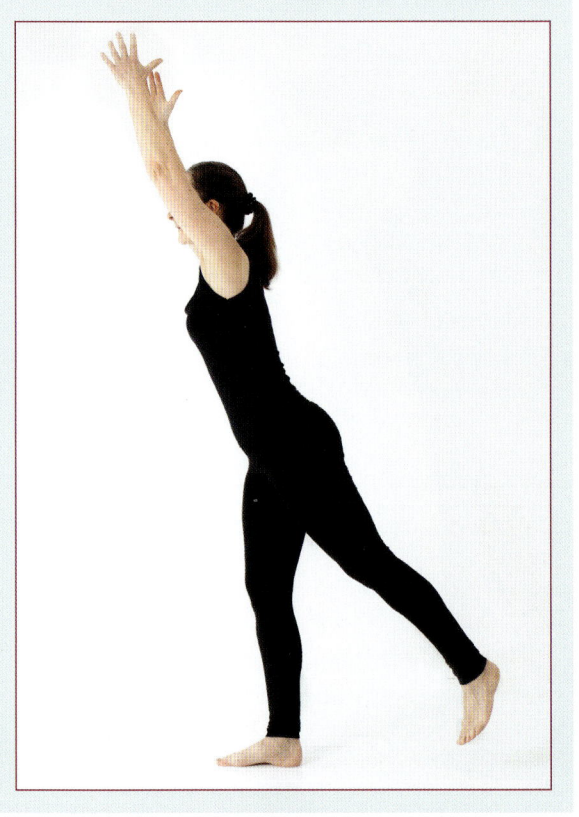

Crescent lunge

I am lucky to have only average back-bending available to my body, and am not able to make the kind of extremely extended shape I often see in yoga teachers advertising their classes, but still I am uncomfortable in the first image.

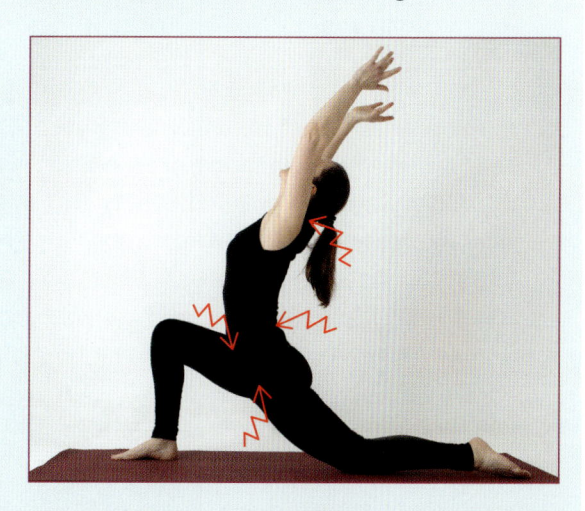

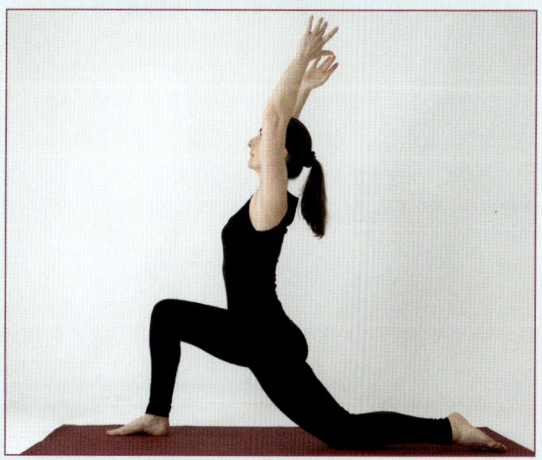

1) Notice a collapsed flaring of the front of the back-leg hip, impingement of the front-leg hip, and though it may not look particularly dramatic, a lumbar extension that for me felt isolated in a couple of vertebrae, and also pressure on an overextended neck.

Rather than dropping the hips, if you consider offering downward pressure through the feet, or drawing the front foot and back knee toward each other (inducing isometric contraction) and a toning of the ligamentous support structure of the hip joints (like a sort of bandha in the back hip) you may also notice a general sense of upward tone in the whole body; a sense of readiness rather than collapse. There may even be a natural engagement of *mula bandha* (the muscular engagement of the pelvic floor sometimes known as "root lock"), which is an aid for pelvic floor tone.

2) In the second version my whole spine is more supported, with extension traveling evenly through all vertebrae, there is less pressure on both labra (the labrum is the cartilage that lines the hip socket), and I feel strong and ready. In the first, I feel physically vulnerable, and not in control.

Feeling the strength of our muscles can make us feel more in control. This is an energy that women in perimenopause greatly value as they can feel at such a loss witnessing the changes that they cannot stop.

Pigeon pose

Before you read on, have a look at these two versions and see if you can see where there might be excess stress, and what you might do to avoid it. Be aware that I am not hypermobile so it's not easy for me to demonstrate the more extreme versions that are not uncommon in yoga studios.

What did you think?

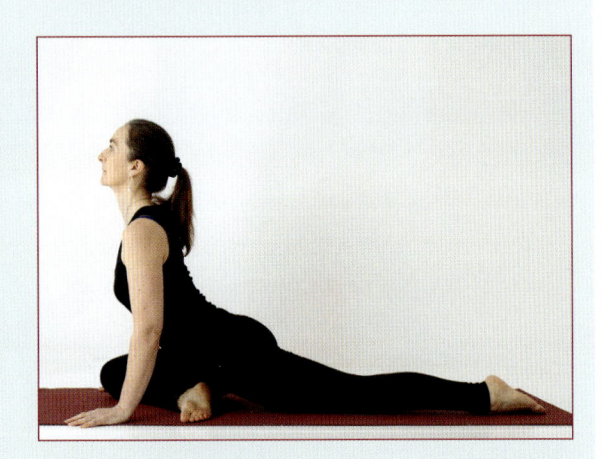

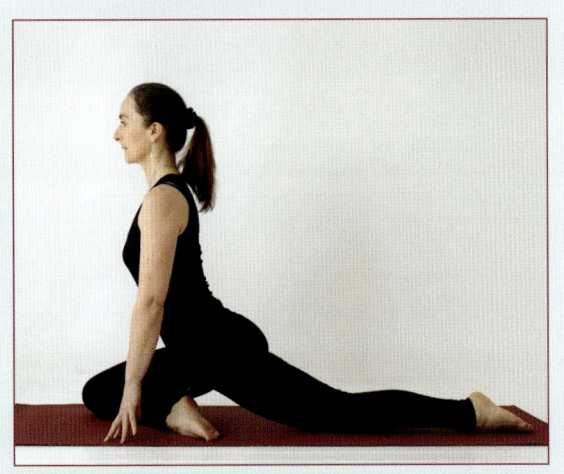

1) In the first version I am using gravity and pushing down (passive stretching) to go lower into the pose. This may be causing pressure of the front of my femoral head into the labrum at the front of my hip socket (back leg), and impingement of my femoral neck into the front of the socket of my front hip. I'm also straining my neck.

    I describe the first version as being like a starfish, splatted on the ocean floor.

2) Instead, I invite you to consider being like a dolphin about to leap out of the water. Press down through the front shin, engage mula bandha. Like zipping up a pair of jeans, draw in and up between the pubic bones and the navel (which is like a light version of *uddiyana bandha*, described on p.145, engage upward at the front of the hip of the back leg (a "hip bandha"). Rise up as if you are going to touch the ceiling with the top of your skull. Feel the strength, active stretch and power of this.

    After some time you can, if the joints feel safe, play with taking a few fingers off the floor or even elevating the hands entirely, but *only* if you can maintain that downward push through the legs, and that upward motion of mula bandha, and are not collapsing your hips. There will be a little wobble and shifting as your muscles get used to this new demand.

Balancing poses

Where osteoporosis is present, standing—and especially balance—poses should be practiced near a wall or sturdy chair to avoid falls. Also, be aware of the possible additional symptoms of vertigo or dizziness.

Make sure to offer and demonstrate a wide range of levels, bringing your student to her individual eustress. Your aim is to help her find the challenge she can work to improve, rather than the challenge that makes her feel out of control, or fall, or become sore or exhausted. Adapted versions shown in these pages may give some of your clients plenty of benefit, more than if they strive without "good form" to "achieve" the full version of the pose. "Good form" is a phrase used in the exercise world to denote performing an exercise well as opposed to unsafely, when control is no longer possible.

All of the balancing poses can be made more useful for meeting the needs of menopausal women by keeping a marginal bend in the standing knee, avoiding taking joints to full range of motion, and lifting the load of the trunk up off the standing femur.

Dancer's pose

Here in dancer's pose, I flex the ankle to activate the back leg and protect the knee. This takes it closer to active than passive stretching because, with activated muscles, I am unable to pull fiercely on the leg and overdo the hip or spine extension.

1) In Dancer, seen on the left, might a micro-bend in the standing knee be safer than locking the joint? Plantar-flexing the ankle could engage some support structures for the raised-leg knee, and taking the backbend through the full spine evenly will reduce any excess pressure on one or two vertebrae.

2) Could the version on the right offer the stretch for some people who don't need a full dancer's pose to feel the front body lengthening, and who value the support of a wall?

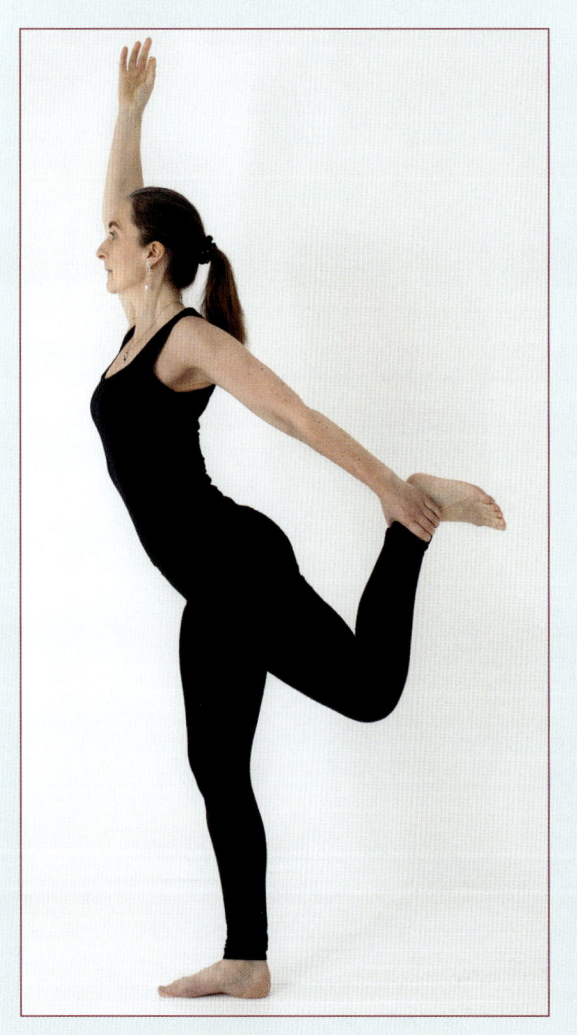

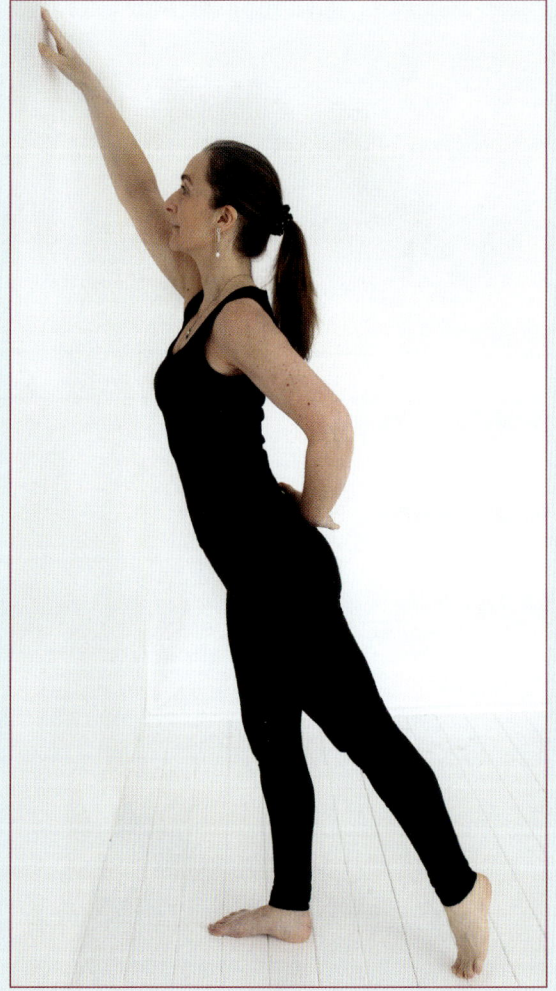

Half moon

1) In this first image my standing knee is locked and I feel a sensation of impingement in my hip.
2) So, to adapt and avoid collapse into the standing-leg hip we can use blocks for the hand, micro-bend the knee, and think of lifting the trunk off the standing leg.

   Encourage use of the legs instead of over-reliance on the arms, by suggesting lightening the load on the hand.

   Using props to bring the floor up to me, my hip is freer, I feel no discomfort, my spine is more able to rotate to take my arm up, and look to the side, giving me a valuable balance challenge. This will make it possible to take my standing hand off the block and be only on my foot. Much more fun!

   One of the graduates of my teacher training said, during her teaching assessment, "There's nothing special about the floor!" I have stolen this phrase to take away the obsession with hands getting to the floor in so many poses.

3) Could this upright version be enough? For some individuals, this more achievable challenge would be preferable to struggling to reach the traditional version of the pose without "good form".

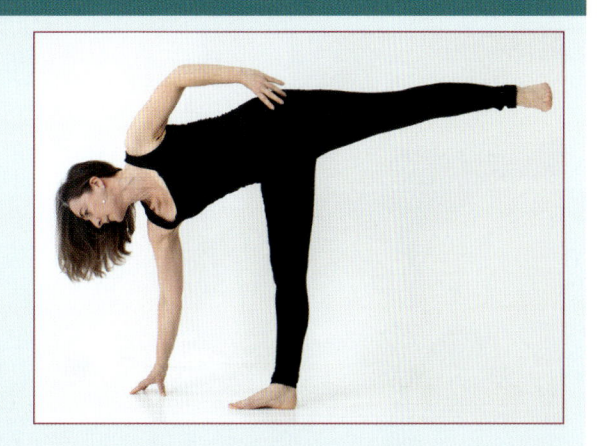

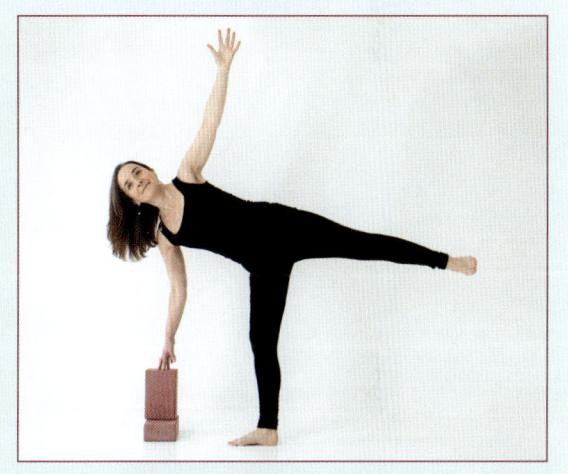

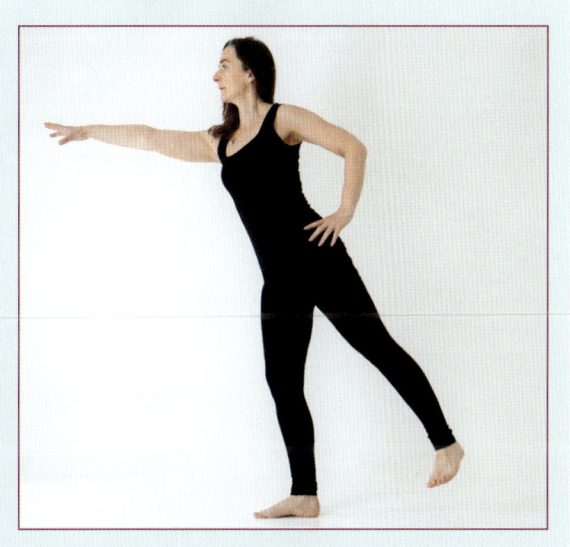

Adding muscular challenge

1) In simple balance poses, or when the student has found their level of manageable challenge, you can add in "press-ups".

2) When steady in any balancing pose, bend the knee a little more on the inhale, and as you exhale, push the foot down to come back up to the starting point. Repeat as often as you feel is challenging but sustainable.

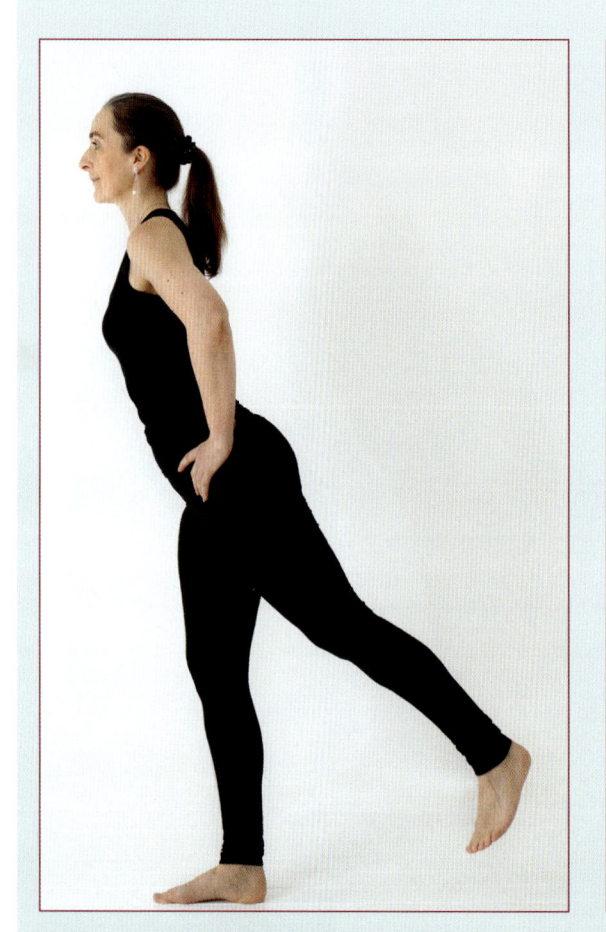

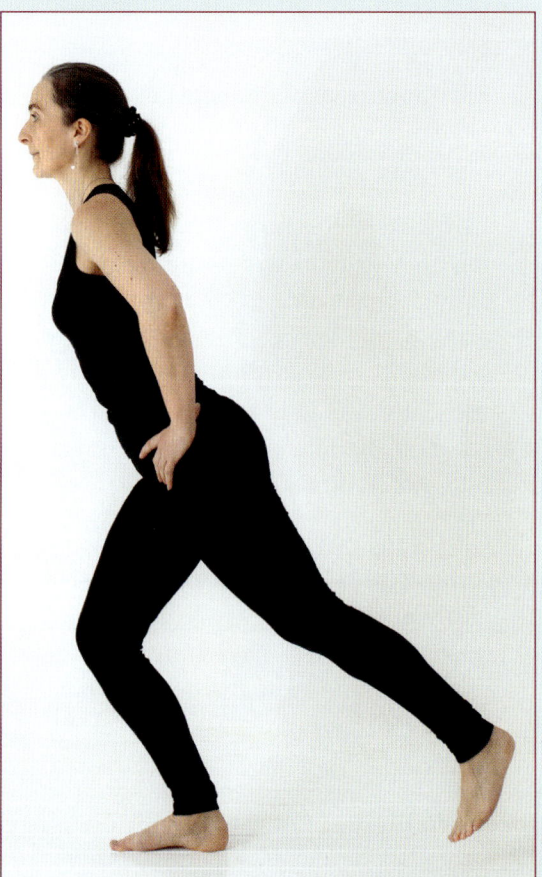

The exercises that follow are a bit more food for thought …

Side-angle pose

1) This is not an uncommon sight in yoga students. It's an obvious strain, with an unintentional twist and flexion of the spine, so it's not safe with osteopenia or osteoporosis.
2) But even in the second image I feel stuck in my front hip, and have no support from my back leg. This is very passive on both legs, and I don't need any core engagement.

   Coming up a little, staying connected to the outer edge of the back foot, tilting at the hip until it reaches full active range of motion, aware of a continuity from my back foot, through the leg across the core and through my top arm, I am aligned enough to elevate my bottom arm, which makes demand on my core.

3) In the first two images, this arm position would not be possible. In fact, you will notice that in offering this arm position, many students will naturally self-adjust to this more functional spine position—they have no choice because of the weight of the lower arm!

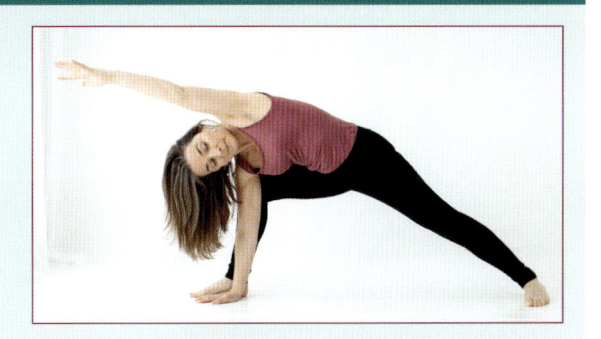

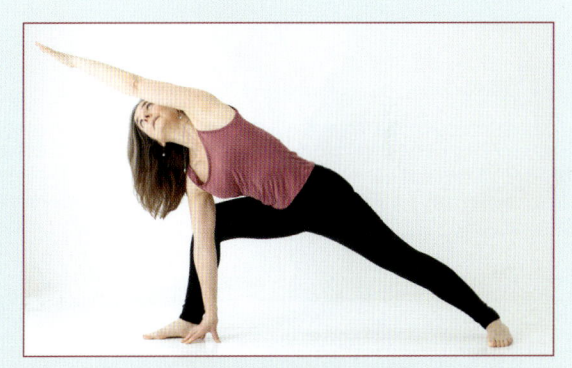

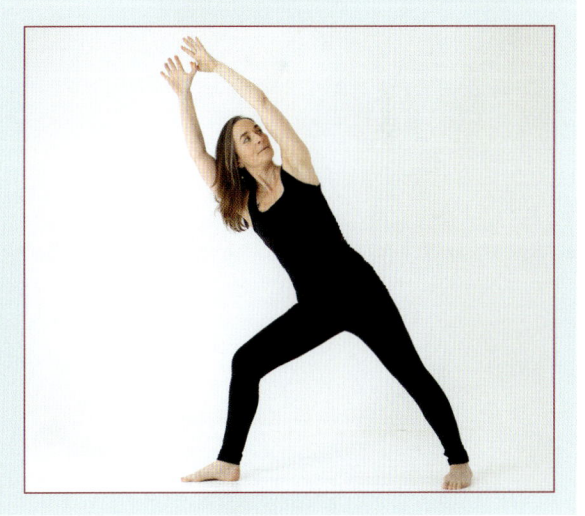

88 YOGA FOR MENOPAUSE AND BEYOND

Intense side-stretch pose

1) In the image on the right this is too intense! With a hyperextended knee, unsafe spine, not only for osteoporosis but also for hamstring and lower back injury risk. I did myself a lot of lower back damage in this pose in the past.

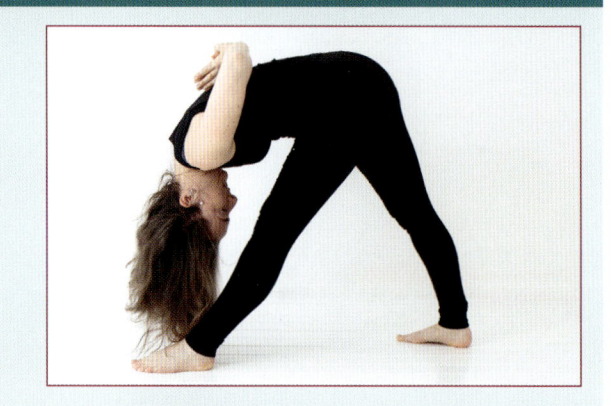

2) How many reasons can you think of, having read this far, why this second version might be better for many women in perimenopause and beyond?

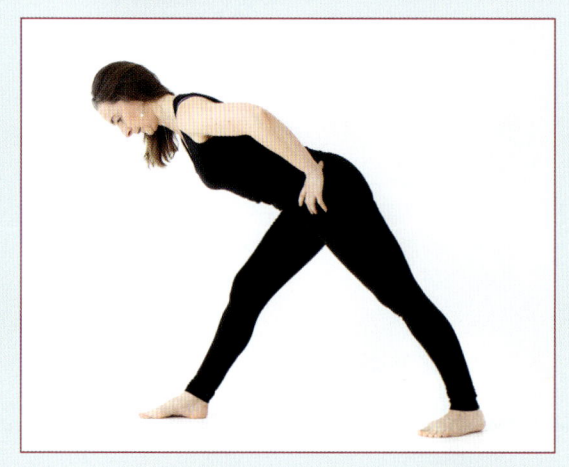

E) REST TIMES, REVALUED

Much as we need the positive stress on our tissues detailed in the last section, it's my belief that restorative yoga is the greatest resource within this tradition for the relief of the fatigue, stress, and self-punishment that can be a great burden in the stages of menopause and contributors to the exacerbation of its symptoms.

Restorative postures, supported Yin yoga practices, and indeed Yoga Nidra, may be places where a woman can feel she is being proactive in rest, rather than feeling guilty for taking time out doing nothing. What I love about many restorative postures is that they can be done without warm-up and give options to simultaneously meditate, deep breathe, or even ... nap!

I truly hope you will transmit to your students the value of rest, especially for women who are sleeping badly, or have other contributors to an overwrought nervous system.

One of the easiest adjustments to a class structure that I teach is to add a restorative pose in addition to shavasana toward the end of a class, or to offer a long restorative as an alternative to shavasana.

In this section I will detail just some of the many restorative and Yin postures that may be useful, and some options for touch, assuming the desire and permission of your students. There are so many possibilities that you will already know, so do explore further.

I include postures from Yin yoga in my teaching, but with an adaptation. Because of what I spoke of regarding passive stretching at end of range of movement, where I use any poses that have come to be associated with Yin over the last few decades, you will see they are generously propped, so that they tend to follow the restorative yoga advice to have every joint supported, and to avoid the pressure of gravity taking the body further into passive stretch.

If any intensity is felt, it should be mild and easeful, and broad over a large area, rather than isolated intensity in one spot or line. The Yin yoga principle of learning to "sit with discomfort" is a valuable one in some ways, but to my mind we as a race, and women in the stages of menopause, have sufficient discomforts to learn to sit with. We don't need to impose further physical risk or stress on our bodies to learn a lesson.

In each of the postures, skilled touch may be offered, with active permission. This touch is not in order to indicate to the practitioner how she could be better positioned or how she ought to relax more. It is to offer a sense of supportive, nurturing care that may subtly release the body into greater ease through suggestions to tissue to relax. Or this touch is simply offered because touch can feel healing and invoke the feel-good hormones.

The hands-on techniques I use and teach are an amalgamation of Thai massage, the Puja Method of Sue Flamm, and the Alexander technique.

Reclining cobbler

Many restorative poses may be of great benefit during perimenopause, but I feel this is the queen of them. This pose affects your whole spine, the fascia of which connects to your internal organs. With the spine in extension, the fascia is mobilized, and blood flow goes anywhere that moves or is taken out of its habitual pattern.

Given that the fascia at the lumbar spine connects to the intestines via the peritoneum, which segues into the mesentery (tissue that connects the small intestine to the abdominal wall), we can reasonably assume a greater flow of all the necessary fluids to and from these viscera.

The back bend also affects the tissue between the ribs and may stimulate diaphragmatic breathing, all of which will move the internal organs, increasing blood flow. As we have seen, organ health is important during this time.

The choice to expose the chest may show our nervous system that we're not afraid, even though we may be feeling anxious, and with a little deep breathing, relaxing the jaw and pelvic floor, we can stimulate the all-important parasympathetic nervous system. If we can do this in an energetically challenging situation, in the safe and trusted environment of a yoga class, that may be a learning to take into daily life. But not if it's too physically or emotionally challenging, because then we are ignoring the signals from our brain that there is something unsafe about this, and if we do that, the brain will not trust us. You will learn how important this is in the section on brain health.

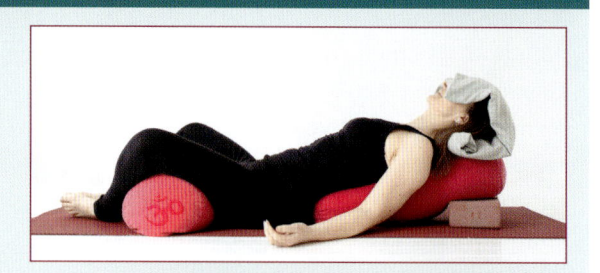

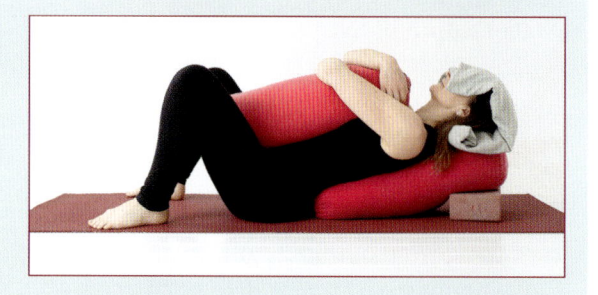

This posture requires support for a lot of joints, and please support them generously so that, even if it feels like a challenge to be so physically exposed, the body is not physically in danger of pain or strain or over-stretch. Also offer options to induce greater emotional ease, like that shown in the second image above.

Options for touch: A gentle holding and then tucking under of the shoulder blades; gentle pressure-point to the shoulders; a holding of the back of the head, with a little optional lengthening gesture to the back of the neck, and/or face and jaw massage.

Meridians: Liver/gall bladder, heart/small intestine, lung/large intestine, kidney/bladder.

Osteoporosis: No contraindications as long as all bones and joints are supported.

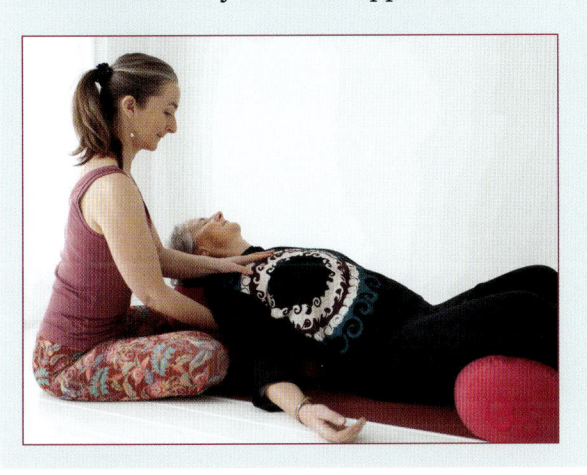

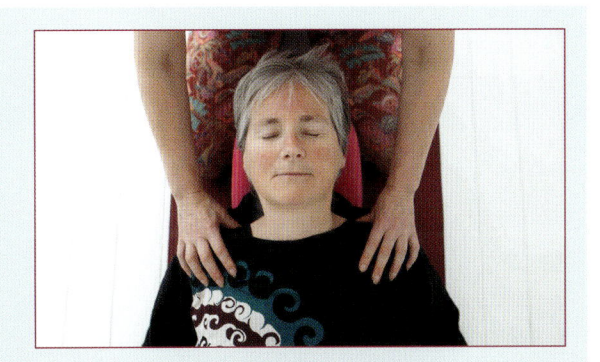

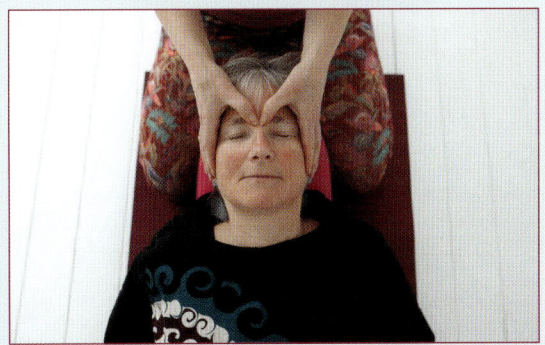

Child's pose

I find this pose a beautiful path to finding our center during menopause. It gives us permission to withdraw from the world at a time when other people's normal demands can be very overwhelming, and can exacerbate symptoms like acopia, fatigue, anxiety, low self-esteem, and more.

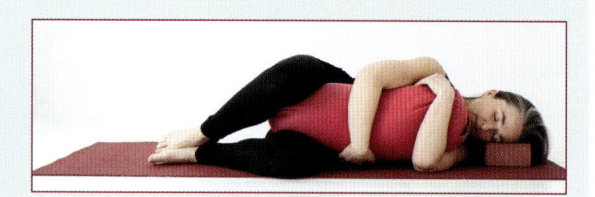

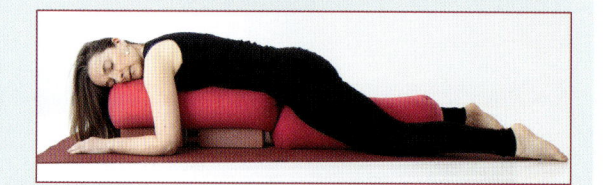

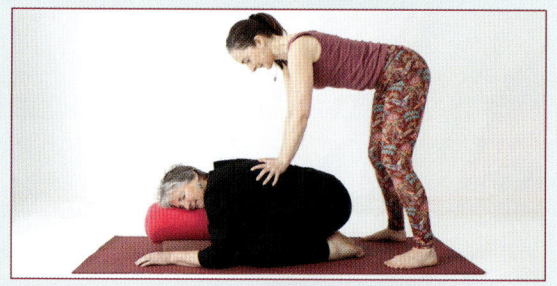

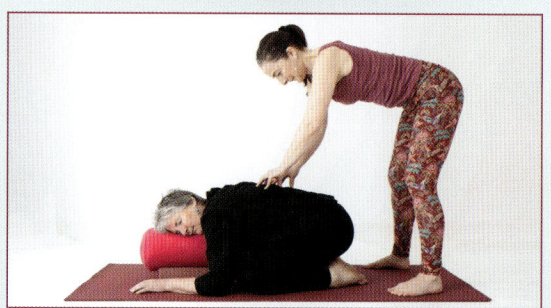

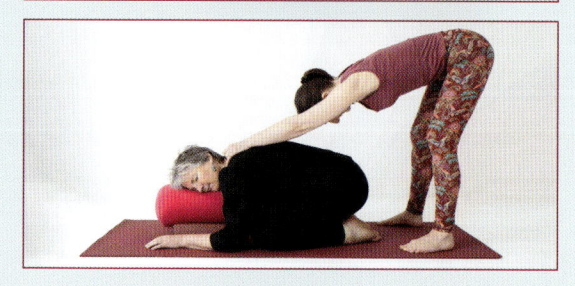

1) I'm putting this hip, knee, ankle and osteoporosis friendly version, and this side-lying one here first because I like to give adjusted postures as much validity as the traditional ones. And it feels lovely!
2) In the second option, make sure that the student's lower abdomen is on the higher bolster; if it's not, this becomes an unintentional back bend. This option is perfect for those with achy hips and/or knees.

Options for touch:
Gentle, symmetrical downward pressure on the pelvis, the lower ribs, and then on the shoulder blades; pressure-point massage on tops of shoulders; "walking" hands down either side of the spine.

Meridians: Depending on the leg position, stomach and spleen (if thighs are compressed), liver (if knees are wide), and kidney.

Osteoporosis: Use the extended leg version as that creates very little rounding of the spine. Don't sell the pose as a back stretch, or clients who don't have the knees under may feel short-changed. (There is an osteoporosis-friendly unsupported child's pose in Chapter 4 a). Keep hands-on pressure gentle.

Some favourite restoratives

Most people need to elevate the pelvis to ensure the possibility of this movement coming from the hips. Most also need support under the knees. If the backs of the knees actually touch the floor, those joints will become hyperextended as we lean forward, so they need supports under them, and if the knees are off the floor, the gap should be filled, in accordance with the restorative principle that no joint should be hanging in space.

This is not the case in the option which has the soles of the wide-spaced feet on the floor (here on the right). In that instance, the feet will adequately support the knees.

Many of my students find this really soothing, as they hug the bolster or rest into it. But very many people can't manage this at all adequately, and in that case, wide legs up the wall with a bolster or chair supporting the outside of each leg would be a nice option, especially if there was also a bolster lying on the front of their trunk to hug.

Here we will feel a considerable connection to the inner thighs (and perhaps activation of the liver meridians that are located there). It stimulates the hips and the backs of the legs also, and is an easy one to achieve after exercise. It is potentially a good pre-sleep de-stressor, not least because it's upright, so your student is less likely to fall asleep just before bed, when a nap can be disastrous for dropping off for the night shortly after!

Options for touch: A press down with the thumbs along the tops of the shoulders.

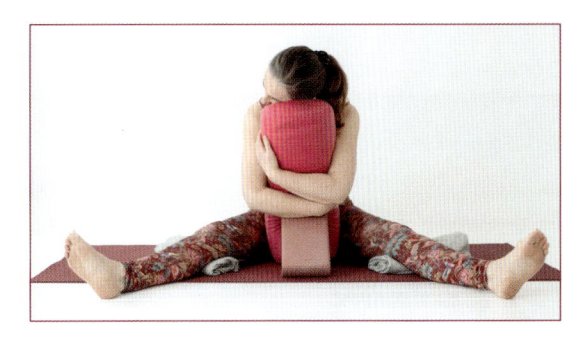

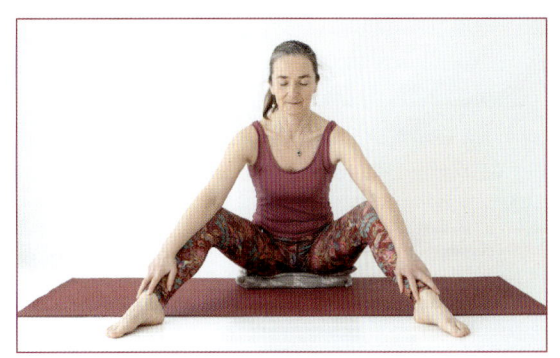

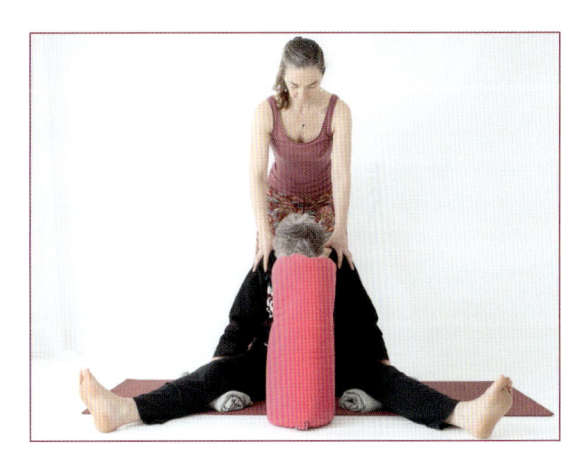

Meridian: Liver/gall bladder.

Osteoporosis: Allow little or no flexion in the spine by elevating the pelvis, not going so far over, ensuring the entire front of the trunk is supported (lean the bolster against a chair to discourage all students from the ego-push to go further forward).

Inversion options

1) Very gentle inversion, but with significant impact on the upper spine, shoulders and neck. It's very important that a natural curve is maintained in the back of the neck by encouraging the chin to lift away from the chest a little before relaxing.
2) This pose may be too much for the lower back for many, so, inserting a folded blanket under the lumbar spine can help, or sliding upward so there is just one bolster, which is only under the pelvis (in the second image).
3) All options can be done with legs resting up the wall or on a chair, and with or without the elevated hips and arms.

4) In this last image, in the Sloth, encourage the limbs to float rather than stretch. If hip mobility doesn't allow verticality of the legs without abdominal effort, use the wall.

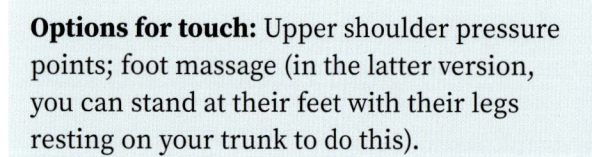

Options for touch: Upper shoulder pressure points; foot massage (in the latter version, you can stand at their feet with their legs resting on your trunk to do this).

Meridians: Lung (which in traditional Chinese medicine TCM is paired with the large intestine) and heart (paired with the small intestine).

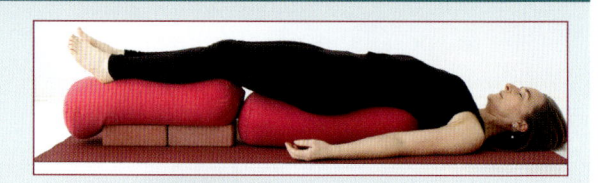

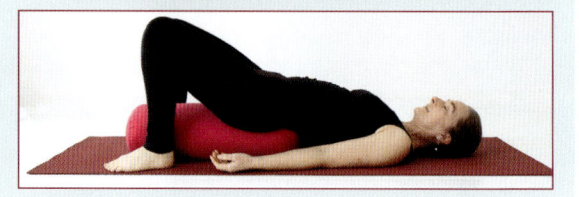

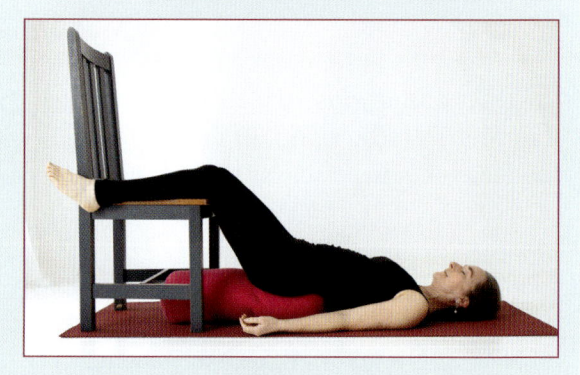

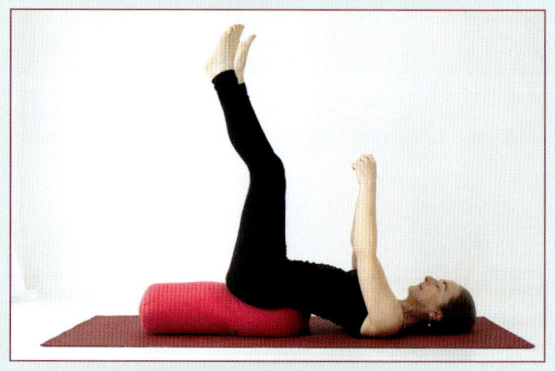

Osteoporosis: Neck flexion should be kept to a minimum, perhaps by letting the head slope back on a folded blanket, or by sliding upward off the bolster a little more to reduce the neck angle.

Twisted deer

1 & 2) Asymmetrical twists can be hard on the lower back. This pressure may be relieved by simply bringing the knees together (second image). Once the spine has settled toward the twist, you may be able to encourage further movement for the neck by turning the head away from the knees.

We're stimulating movement and compression of the gut here, and we know keeping the bowels moving is important. We're also stimulating the accessory breathing mechanisms and mobilizing potentially stuck tissue in the upper back. It's also a stimulus for hip flexors, psoas muscles and abdominals if the top leg is reaching back.

Options for touch: Gentle downward pressure on both shoulder blades; gentle diagonal space-making pressure between the diagonally opposite sides of the pelvis and the shoulder blade area.

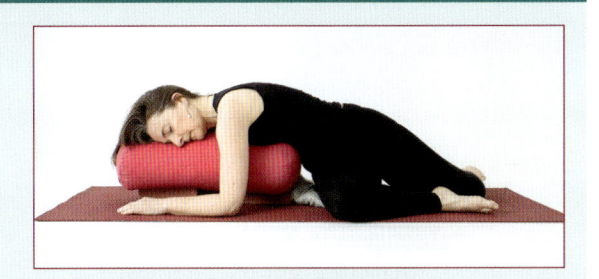

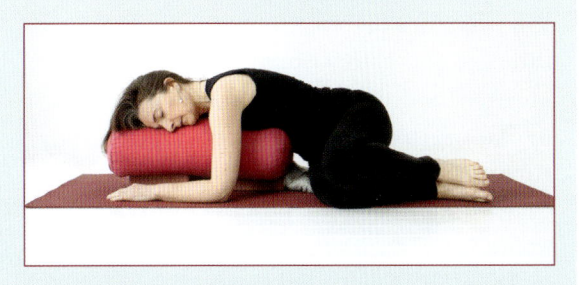

Meridians: Stomach/spleen.

Osteoporosis: Keep the spine long (minimize rounded back by elevating the bolster). Keep knees together so the twist is more in the thoracic spine. Don't turn the head away from the knees. Keep the hands-on pressure very soft.

A note on meridians

I have mentioned meridians above because they are a central aspect of Yin yoga, but I share here only my knowledge in this regard from my own education in Yin yoga, having not trained in traditional Chinese medicine (TCM).

However, I do so to point out that during Yin practices there is an opportunity to indicate gently to women the importance of organ health. In addition, the elements of TCM with regard to the organ/emotion relationship can be a really helpful way to introduce conversation in your classes about the nature of normal versus chronic or knee-jerk emotional states.

I would recommend you research further. But here is a little shorthand to get you started:

Meridians	Imbalanced	Balanced
Kidney/Bladder	Fear	Wisdom
Liver/Gall Bladder	Anger	Compassion
Spleen/Stomach	Anxiety	Calm
Lungs/Large Intestine	Sadness	Courage
Heart/Small Intestine	Hate	Love

There are nuances, of course, and the emotions listed under "Imbalanced" are only considered problematic if they are chronic or habitual, and not a reasonable response to a particular stimulus. It's important to recognize that a woman's emotional reactions are not always just a symptom of hormone shifts. It may be in fact that the hormonal shifts have made clear that stressors she has tolerated for too long should no longer be tolerated. This can be a huge and immensely empowering perspective shift, especially for women who are very judgmental of their new emotional states. I hope you will use any opportunity you can to indicate to women that, for example, their rage may be well founded or their impatience a very reasonable reaction to too much demand.

The value of an intuitive, inquiring, self-accepting, emotional approach to yoga is in developing an ability to feel, then rightly analyze, what arises in the layers of our being, and from that place of knowing, come to a response that is in sympathy with the stimulus.

> *Between stimulus and response there is a space, and in that space lies our power to choose our response, and in our response lies our growth and freedom.*
> —Viktor Frankl

Yoga Nidra

There are very few elements of yoga that cannot be used, and enhanced, to add to your teaching toolkit, and to your students' targeted supports. Yoga Nidra is a rich resource, and its simplest form, as traditionally taught, is just perfect. But it is open to a wonderful variety of nuances too!

The body scan can help bring your client toward deeper interoception and thereby discernment, so that she can begin to know which of her sensations are normal and non-threatening and what may be medically significant and need investigation and treatment.

The awareness of opposite sensations in the body—weight and lightness, heat and cold, restlessness and calm, etc.,—may create a sense of the possibility of choice of sensation (remembering coolness when hot-flashing, for example) or at the very least a reminder that nothing stays, and that uncomfortable and comfortable sensations will come and go. The choice of what sensations you help them explore, and what common visualizations of Yoga Nidra you use, can be made according to the needs of individual clients.

The sensing of opposite emotions may be a technique that can offer "calm abidance" (known as *shamata* in the Buddhist tradition) of the opposing emotions of grief and anticipation, lack of control and freedom, or strength and disempowerment that a woman will be experiencing. Be very careful here as to the sensibilities in the room, of course, the length of time you have been with a group, how easily you think you can hold them, etc. These may be the kind of depths you can only explore on a retreat or with a very familiar long-standing group.

Shavasana

During shavasana, there is one more option for touch I would like to offer you, while reminding you to be careful that you don't exhaust yourself. In offering Yin/restorative two-hour sessions with touch, which I call Yin Safe Hands, I found that I could give touch in two postures when I had a group of up to 15–30 mini massages! (At first I tried to do it for every posture and became exhausted.)

Thai foot massage

This is from my training in Thai massage.

(I usually drape a light blanket over the feet to protect myself from varieties of grubbiness picked up off a studio floor, but bare feet were better for the images here.)

1. Begin by pressing the sides of your palms downward on their inner heels. Hold for 5–10 seconds.

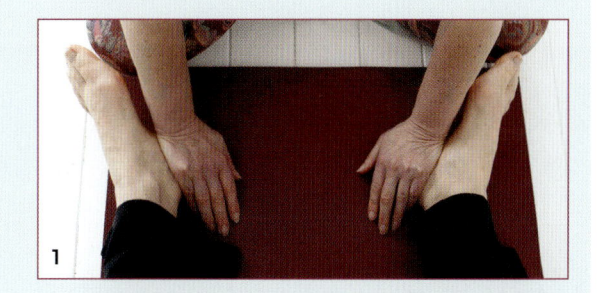

2. Then, beginning at the center of the instep as close to the heel as possible, press in with your thumbs while gently pulling the rest of the foot toward you (as if aiming to point the feet).

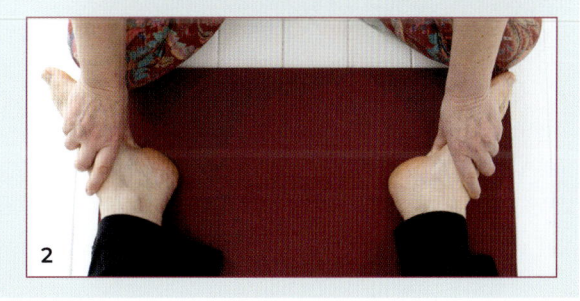

3. Then press your thumbs into the center of the inner side of the sole of the foot, in line with the big toe, also pulling the toes gently toward you with the entirety of the fingers and palms.

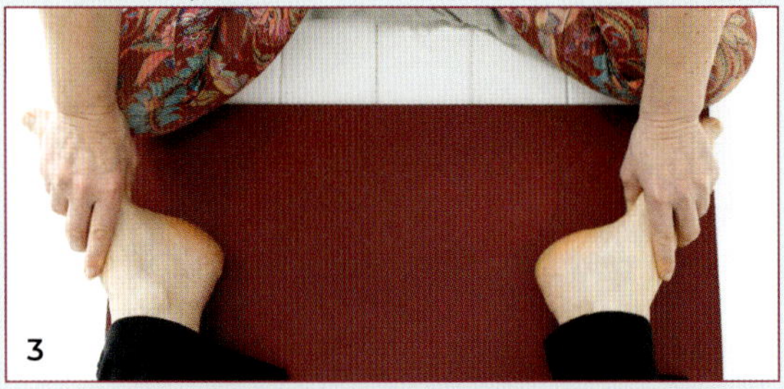

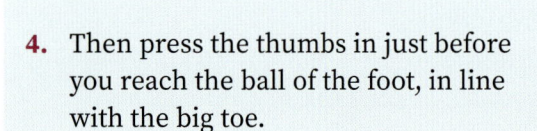

4. Then press the thumbs in just before you reach the ball of the foot, in line with the big toe.

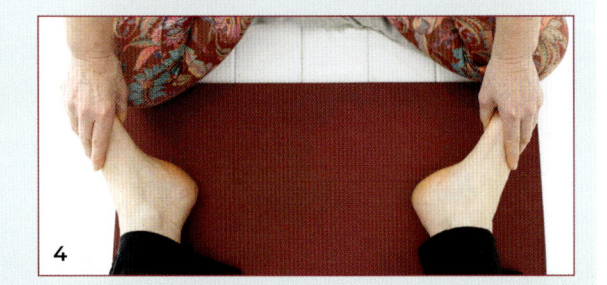

5. Next, use your thumb on the ball of the foot at the base of the big toe to press and circle, massaging the knuckle of the big toe.

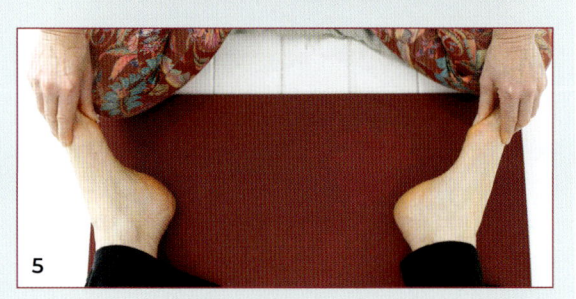

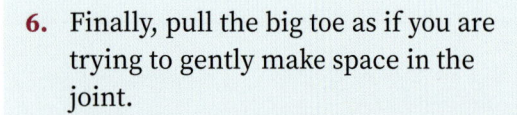

6. Finally, pull the big toe as if you are trying to gently make space in the joint.

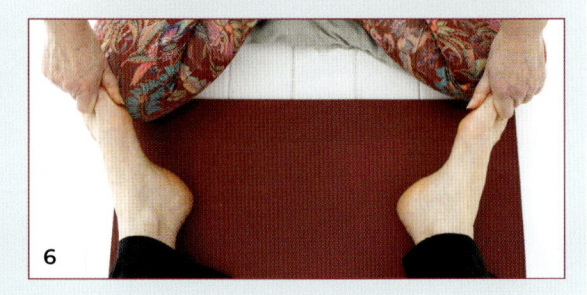

Repeat steps 2 to 6, starting at the center near the heel, and following the line up the instep toward each toe. This means you will perform the instep massage five times. If you are short of time, you could do it just three times, but be sure to give each toe its satisfying pull.

During restorative or Yin poses and/or shavasana, you have a great opportunity to offer readings, meditations, breath practice, and ... silence. As always when teaching yoga, particularly to women

Finish with the heel press again.

Oh, how lucky our students are!

whose life stage may be bringing them into unusual levels of emotional vulnerability, it's essential to remind yourself of trauma-sensitive teaching.

F) MEDITATION AND BREATH, RENEWED

As teachers, we all have our approaches to meditation and breath work, just as we do to all aspects of yoga. Below, I hope to offer you new ways of using these practices to more specifically benefit your midlife students.

If meditation is something that your student can approach without the expectation or aim to "improve" herself (or to achieve ultimate and enduring calm and therefore be inevitably frustrated!), it can be a great and accessible tool for her own use. Likewise, Pranayama.

In my decades of teaching I have taught Pranayama and meditation, assuming everyone was enjoying them, only to realize, when I became more interested in discovering people's *actual* individual experience, that many women were frustrated in meditation by a perceived lack of ability to still the mind or stay focused, or to achieve mastery of, or comfort in, complex breath practices.

An essential aim in supporting women in the stages of menopause is to help them to come toward a simpler way of being, or to reduce their load so that they can enjoy kinder expectations of themselves than before, as their bodies begin naturally to slow down and demand rest.

Seated positions

Sitting for prolonged periods with deep knee or hip flexion for meditation or breath work, can be fine—until we get up.

Even with my years of yoga practice, and being comfortable *while* seated in a more classical pose, I find my hips and knees can struggle to come back to mobility and comfort afterward, especially if I am teaching a lot of classes or a retreat.

In the following four images are some sitting options I really encourage you to try yourself, and to offer and normalize for your students. Remember that they will most likely want to emulate you, so please choose, even just in class, the posture that supports the person least able to get comfortable in the classical sitting postures.

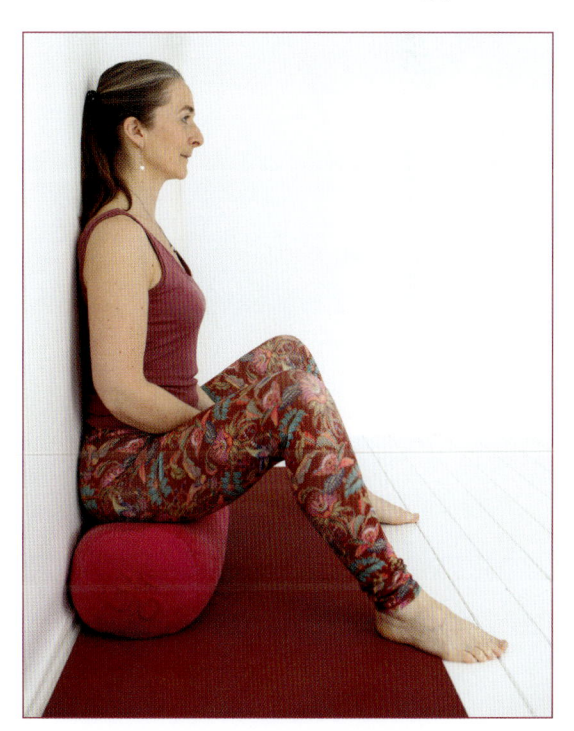

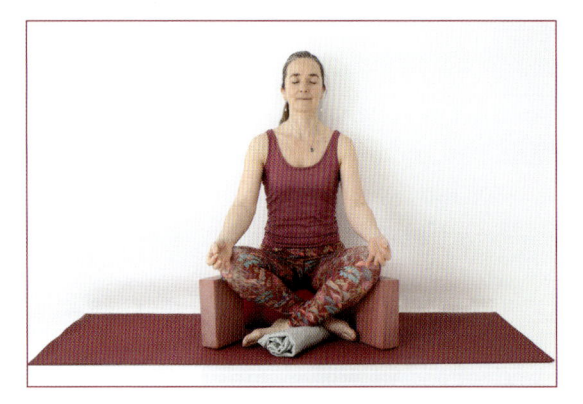

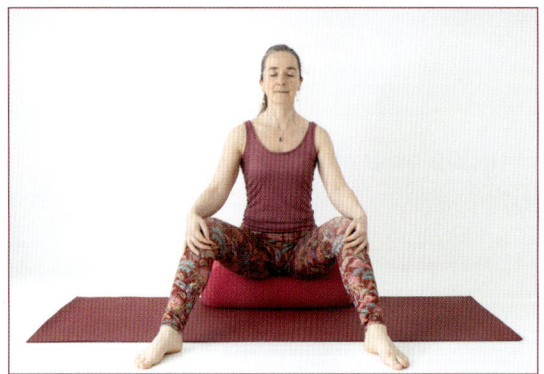

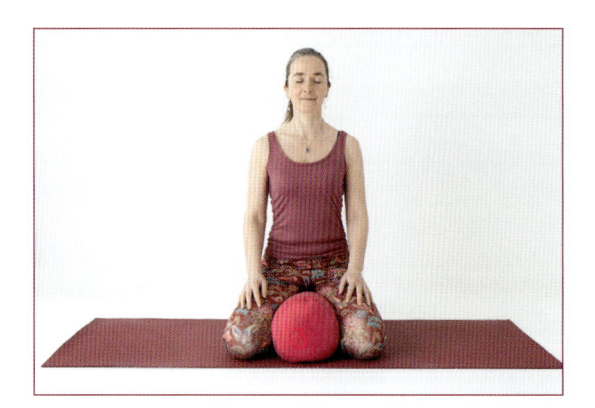

Pranayama

I don't recommend throwing a lot of complicated pranayama practices into the mix, but rather helping your student to focus on habituating something really simple that she can use at any time, perhaps as an accessible tool in a moment of acute anxiety, even in company or in the car.

You may read in articles that some practices like bhastrika and kapalabhati should be avoided because they are "heating". This would not be a reason I would avoid them. In my experience, no pranayama has ever induced a hot flash, unless it is because that practice is very stressful for the individual.

The mechanism of hot flashes is not fully known, and is clearly complex, and we certainly don't have studies about such practices inducing hot flashes. But in beginners I tend to avoid anything that can be difficult to achieve and therefore affect a woman's self-esteem, or that aren't fun or pleasurable. Kapalabhati can be tricky to master for some, and therefore difficult to enjoy.

However, you read about some benefits of these pranayama in Chapter 2, so depending on your aim, most things have a place. In fact, it may be beneficial to offer them. For starters, trying to avoid "heating" practices may only serve to reinforce the idea of a hot flash as something awful to be avoided at all costs, whereas, as will be discussed in Chapter 5 where I look at symptoms, changing our relationship with these moments may be more sustainable, given how many years they may stay with us. So, perhaps we could tempt that hot flash—though I would love to hear if you meet anyone who can actually induce one through a breath practice. If you do, help her to notice that she is brave enough to experience the sensation rather than run from it.

You may also be interested in teaching sitali and sitkari pranayama, despite my critique of their commonly claimed benefits in Chapter 2. The cool sensation in the mouth may be a pleasure to feel during a hot flash, just as the cool air on your skin may be when you shed a garment or get out into a cooling breeze.

I enjoy teaching ujjayi pranayama, and even beginners find it very soothing. Given that humming and chanting stimulate the vocal folds, and that this in turn stimulates the vagus nerve to support the parasympathetic response, I expect there is a similar value to ujjayi, given that the vocal folds are also involved.

Breathing from a research-based perspective

For perimenopause, ease, achievability, and feasibility of use outside a class or dedicated practice is paramount. Regular yogis may be perfectly comfortable with any or all Pranayama. This may or may not change for them in the stages of menopause.

Like many elements of yoga, some breath practices have been taken and researched under names other than those yoga might give them. Let's use that research!

"Paced breath," which is basically diaphragmatic breathing of five to six breaths per minute, has been seen in clinical trials to have positive effects on the duration and severity of hot flashes (Sood et al, 2013).

Practicing this deep breathing for 15 minutes twice per day (and to a lesser extent, once per day) was seen in that study to have effective impact on hot flashes, yet there were also people who benefitted from pausing twice for 15 minutes to breathe normally. Yet again, we make no promises, because another study (Huang et al, 2015) found that results were better for the group listening to relaxing music than for the paced breathing group. As always, we see there are no definitive answers. But this is a breath practice for which there is enough research evidence for reputable menopause organizations to add it to their recommendations. So we should too!

Another technique researched and recognized by the medical community is "boxed breath": breathing in—holding—exhaling—holding, for equal counts. These are simple, achievable pranayama practices you can easily share. I adopted two lovely alternatives to the more grim instructions of Inhale, hold, exhale, hold, from two separate teachers whose names, unfortunately, I can't recall in order to give them credit. One is "watercolor breath":

> *Imagine you have some beautiful watercolor paper, paints, and a brush. As you inhale, visualize yourself painting an upward stroke on the side of the page. As you gently pause, imagine the color sweeping across the top of the page. As you softly exhale, see the beautiful color sweep down the side. As you pause, paint that color across the bottom of the page. Etcetera.*

The other is "seasons breath":

> *As you inhale, picture this as alike to the growth of Spring. As you pause at the top, imagine the fullness of Summer. As you exhale, this is the winding down of Autumn. As you pause, feel the stillness of Winter. Etcetera.*

Apologies and thanks to these two teachers.

The recommendation from the paced breathing study is 15 minutes of breath work, preferably twice per day, but more achievably once, to garner results. This should be balanced with maintaining low demand on your student in her day. Perhaps suggest spacing those 15 minutes out into bite-sized moments in the car, while the kettle boils, or on the toilet!

I often use the following concepts when teaching the "Yes/no" practice in the somatics section. You can add this as she breathes:

> *As you inhale, feel that you can expand upward and outward into community while still connected to the support of the earth. As you exhale, feel yourself aware of the resources in your own center, coming back to your quiet, core connection with yourself.*

Guided meditations

In perimenopause in particular, when women may be more emotionally delicate, more easily triggered, harsher on themselves, and are struggling with how to adapt their perspectives and life to support their changes, I believe guided meditations may be a powerful tool. Below I share some that I love to use in class or with clients. You might find them a useful offering.

Spaces meditation

This may be helpful to women feeling that sense of overwhelm when the demands of family or work colleagues creates a sort of claustrophobia and desire to "escape." Clearly there are pauses as you see fit, and scope for your own words.

> *Preferably sitting, close your eyes if that's comfortable for you, or drop your gaze. Become aware of your body in the room. Be aware of the shape it makes.*
>
> *Be aware of molecules of air around you, and that as you breathe, they shift. Become aware of the space around you that you directly affect.*
>
> *Become aware of more space around you.*
>
> *Allow yourself to expand into that space.*
>
> *Then become aware of the space in front of you. Picture it.*

Then extend your awareness to the wall in front.

Then picture the space beyond the wall into the next room, the garden, or street.

See beyond that to roads, onward over houses, fields, rivers, mountains, towns, fields, roads, all the way to the coast and the sea. (Take your time with these.)

(Repeat this journeying with the spaces behind, to each side, below to the earth's core, and above into the universe.)

Then imagine that you are fashioning a sphere in your hands, made of the substance of that universe.

Then visualize that sphere in the center of your brain.

See the sphere of dark and space in the center of your brain. Give it substance.

Then let the sphere disappear. (Here I usually enter into a silent meditation of between two and 10 minutes, the duration of which I have agreed with the person or group. Many feel that the visualization of the sphere in the brain, and then its disappearance, creates a moment or long moments of spaciousness between thoughts, of that longed-for relief from the chatter.)

Then bring your awareness back to your breath, and feel your breath as a protective glow around you, giving you your own space at all times.

Thank you to Sarah Lo, Yin teacher trainer, who offered me a similar meditation and inspired this little adaptation of mine. What I changed was the image of what would be imagined in the brain. She used an orange, and really encouraged me to visualize its substance. Then it disappeared leaving a space. I found it really effective except that when I taught the meditation, I found the introduction of an orange somehow jarring or comical. So I came up with the sphere fashioned from the universe. So, you see the possibility of personalizing your teaching so that you are comfortable.

Self-advocacy meditation

One of the greatest enemies of a reasonable journey through menopause is the assumption that a woman should maintain productivity in the same way as she did before her hormones began to change. This stops her from being able to see, or to acknowledge, the changing requests from her body. This meditation and the following one may be of help. (Each of these possible scripts would be delivered once you have guided your student into stillness and ease in the body and breath.)

Take a moment to bring into your awareness one or two of the most frequently present effects of your hormonal life at the moment …

What are these symptoms affecting in your day-to-day life? …

When are they most present? …

Think about one or two more …

How do they challenge you, and when are they most problematic? …

Think of one of those struggles …

When is it lessened? …

And another … When is it less intense? …

What would these struggles suggest to you if they could ask you for what they need to be able to ease? …

Think of someone in your life who you love …

Picture them with a similar struggle …

What would you say if they asked you for help? …

Picture yourself in your struggle …

Ask yourself: "What would make this easier for you?" …

What is your menopause asking of you? …

Can you allow your body to receive the help or the adjustments to your life that it is asking for?

Expectations meditation

The following meditation, which was inspired by my wise friend and colleague Petra Fulham, might be delivered after conversation in a one-to-one setting so that you can address specific frustrations spoken about by the individual or a selection of concerns raised in a group.

A client of mine, who is a yoga teacher, was really struggling with regard to the following: her changing body shape, keeping on top of a very strict dietary regimen, her need to be constantly practicing to "keep ahead" of her students, her tiredness, her impatience with her family, and the mess of her house. Her house was very tidy. She had two small kids, and when they were at school she tidied, cleaned and prepared the time-consuming organic, vegan, low-carb diet she was choosing. When she did yoga, it was only with an eye to developing her teaching. She never rested because there was always something to be done.

Having first talked to her on a fact-based level about the changing needs of a woman's body (particularly the need for more rest and more regular and rich nutrition), the relationship of excess exercise and low-calorie diets to high cortisol (and thereby, weight gain), the stress that maintaining high standards can add to the sense of overwhelm (despite one's impression that those are "healthy options") and the value of simplifying some of the demands we place on ourselves (in order to protect our brain and body from the effects of stress), I brought her through this meditation. Of course, you would adapt it, depending on your client's/student's life.

Take a moment to ask yourself, What are my expectations of myself with regard to my teaching? …

> Then consider:
>
> Are they achievable given my current circumstances, being aware of my other demands from family, my health challenges, my finances?
>
> Am I flexible about these expectations—by which I mean, if I don't achieve what I expect of myself on any given day, will I be okay with that, or will it knock me back?
>
> Are these expectations sustainable in the medium- to long-term? Are these expectations kind to my body, heart, and mind?
>
> Now ask: What are my expectations of myself with regard to my food choices? ... Are they achievable in my current circumstances? Am I flexible about them? Are they sustainable? Are they kind?
>
> What are my expectations of myself with regard to my body? ... Are they achievable? Am I flexible about them? Are they sustainable in the long term? Are they kind?
>
> What are my expectations of myself with regard to my relationships? ... Are they achievable? Am I flexible about them? Are they sustainable in the long term? Are they kind?
>
> What are my expectations of myself with regard to my productivity each day? ... Are they achievable? Am I flexible about them? Are they sustainable in the long term? Are they kind?
>
> Can you notice one small thing in your life that you could allow yourself to relax around to make a space where you can sit and do absolutely nothing? ... Not meditate, not do yoga, not consciously breathe, not plan, but perhaps sit and stare into space ...
>
> How does it feel in your body to imagine yourself sitting down and doing absolutely nothing?

What do you think of her expectations of herself?

The thing is, the majority of women in the Western world will be endeavoring to uphold demands like this—and more—at a time when our organism is asking us to slow down. It's not a case of surrendering to aging, or letting go of our brilliance, our skills, our passions, and capabilities. It's about adjusting our habits, advocating for ourselves to get the supports we need so that we can protect brain function, cardiovascular health, bone health, and more—the damage to which is a very real risk, a risk which is heightened by stress and fatigue.

This is some of the deeply heartening response I had from her a month later:

> Thank you so much for putting this meditation together, it's amazing the effect already. I am taking things a lot more easily, building in rest, not being

so uptight with food choices and today I went swimming for my non-yoga-related activity. How hard can it be to give myself a little rest and pleasure every day? I have asked the boys and my husband to get me a weighted blanket for Xmas, so that is going to become my daily treat ... It's such a relief to feel it's ok to slow down, that it's normal to not be able or feel like doing what I used to do ... and to listen to and trust what my body is trying to tell me is energizing and uplifting.

Subsequently, she took my teacher training and is now running workshops in New York for women in perimenopause and beyond. We yoga teachers find it hard not to turn our passions into care of others!

In any meditations you choose, keep in mind *ahimsa*, *metta*, and *karuna* (non-violence, loving-kindness, and compassion) with regard to the self. Your student may have spent her adult life minding everyone around her. Now she needs minding, and she is the person who can begin to notice that need for herself, begin to give herself more kind care, and hopefully then begin to expect and demand it from those around her.

Perspective shifts

During meditation or restorative postures or shavasana, you can offer some perspective shifts as guided meditations of your own making. It may be helpful, in order to convince your participants of their deserved place in our society as honored, wise, and valuable elders, to offer these considerations:

In our youth-idolizing Western culture, menopause can seem like an ending. However, in many cultures, menopause is a time of new respect and freedom for women. Mayan women, for example, tend to look forward to menopause because with it comes a progressive change in status within their communities and, in turn, a feeling of freedom. When women from some cultures cross into menopause, they become known as "wise women" or spiritual leaders and hold a place of power in their communities.

In a study into symptom severity and relationship impacts of menopause, the authors saw fewer symptoms in countries where aging is not seen as negatively as in the US, Canada, and the UK where symptoms are reportedly worse (Minkin et al, 2015). In an interview for Reuters, Dr Minkin said:

> *In societies where age is more revered and the older woman is the wiser and better woman, menopausal symptoms are significantly less bothersome. Where older is not better, many women equate menopause with old age, and symptoms can be much more devastating.*
> (Rapaport, 2015)

There are many women writing beautiful things about the menopausal woman and her journey whom you can find on the World Wide Web to inspire you, or whom you can quote in guided meditations if their language seems useful to you for what you are hoping to give to your students. You are, of course, welcome to read/quote passages from my writing here or on social media.

I didn't expect to reference Wikipedia in this book but it offers an excellent overview of the fascinating "Grandmother Hypothesis", which is an anthropological view of menopause as an evolutionary step which actually increases the success of the bloodline of that woman.1 In communities where women are involved in the care of their grandchildren, their immediate offspring tend to have more children than when a family does not have the contribution of the grandmother. This increases the number of her genetic offspring. Now, this may not be so important in our overcrowded world, but putting that aside, and given that all species' main drive is to procreate, you can see where the evolutionary benefit might be.

Cognitive behavioral therapy

Let's take a look at CBT, as elements of it can be easily introduced during, or as a preparation for, meditation. It is a talk-therapy technique widely used to alleviate mental health struggles, or struggles that are contributed to by the way we think, largely by changing those thoughts. My interpretation is that, at its heart, it seeks to neutralize thinking, so that a person can avoid adding to their suffering by overlaying it with catastrophic or victimhood thinking. Research has shown that CBT can aid the reduction of some of the common menopausal symptoms.

Unless you are trained in CBT I don't advise you to take your clients on a CBT-based intervention. But when you look at CBT you will notice that a) there is a huge resource any person can look up on the World Wide Web and use without professional help anyway, and b) the concepts and language are very familiar to us all from our training and immersion in yoga.

As I said in Chapter 2, I believe it falls easily under the principles of svadhyaya, ahimsa, satya, and the practice of pratipaksha-bhavana. It is also credible that it fits in with the principles of *brahmacharya* (self-restraint) and *aparygraha* (simplicity and non-attachment).

Much of what we have looked at is essentially CBT. For instance:

- changing the language we use in class to avoid unwitting harm to self-esteem
- bolstering self-esteem by offering achievable, rather than difficult, tasks or practices
- helping women to understand that most of their *symptoms* are passing (as distinct from *health concerns* which will continue to need prevention/minimizing throughout life)
- suggesting a woman looks for pleasurable ways to stay well
- reminding clients that life in our 50s is usually smoother than life in our 40s.

Becoming attached to the story of victimhood in our struggles, or the rights

---

[1] Wikipedia, Grandmother Hypothesis: https://en.wikipedia.org/wiki/Grandmother_hypothesis. Accessed 09.06.23.

and wrongs of other people's ways of doing things, or diving into the depths of catastrophic thinking during, for example, a hot flash, are not in keeping with any of those yogic principles outlined above.

However, and immensely importantly, to imply that women are being self-indulgent or non-yogic by being unable to manage the burden of those seismic shifts would be a cruelty akin to expecting someone to meditate outside in the middle of gale-force winds.

In Chapter 5 a) on p.161, there are details of some of the applications of CBT.

CHAPTER 4

ENHANCING YOGA FOR MENOPAUSE HEALTH

In the last sections, I guided you through ways in which we might re-imagine what we do in most yoga classes and workshops. It may already seem like a considerable shift.

In the three main sections of this chapter I address the three health concerns connected with menopause that are arguably most targetable through yoga: the bones, the brain and the pelvic floor. No tool for one region is without benefits for others.

In this section, and in Chapter 5, I offer nutrition guidance specific to the area being addressed. Please note that, though yoga does have its principles concerning diet, being a yoga teacher does not make us qualified to address an individual's nutritional needs. However, nutrition is such a cornerstone to health that I include it here for you to be aware of in the background. There is nothing to stop you sharing bits of what you learn anecdotally, as long as you are open with your student as to your level of expertise, and make it clear that they shouldn't make any dietary changes without checking with their doctor or a nutritional therapist/functional medicine practitioner, especially if they are on *any* medications or have any current health issues.

A) BONES

The changing biology

Essentially, bone formation (osteogenesis) occurs when the osteoblasts that lie in the bone turn into osteocytes (bone tissue). This happens in balance with the natural breakdown of bone tissue (resorption) until our bones reach peak mass, usually between the ages of 20 and 30, depending on their location in the body. Then the balance shifts and there is more breakdown than growth.

By the time we are entering menopause there may already be osteopenia (low bone mass, which is considered a precursor to osteoporosis), and the risks will continue to rise. Many people think of osteoporosis as a disease of the elderly, but it is quite common for women in their early 50s to have osteopenia or even osteoporosis, and some are diagnosed in their 20s and 30s. Approximately 50% of people in the USA have osteopenia

(Harvard Health, 2021), and women are twice as likely to have osteopenia as men, and four times likelier to have osteoporosis (Rinonapoli et al, 2021).

Given that many women will not have a bone density scan (DEXA) until they suffer a fracture, the proportion of women with osteoporosis may be higher than statistics show. It is sometimes called the "silent disease" because a person may not be aware that they have osteoporosis until they have experienced either a low-impact fracture or a vertebral compression fracture (VCF). This may be why we think it doesn't occur until old age, when balance issues begin to cause more falls and posture changes because of VCFs can cause more chronic rounding of the spine.

Certainly there are more women in your classes than you know, and more than know themselves, who have low BMD, not least because in the five to seven years directly after menopause in particular, there appears to be an accelerated loss of bone mineral density (BMD).

Fractures related to low bone density are thought to be more common in people with osteoporosis than osteopenia. But interestingly, one study showed that people with osteopenia and low body weight had a greater fracture risk than those with osteoporosis (Tomasevic-Todorovic et al, 2018). This points to the need for adjustments to be made for people who have osteopenia, rather than waiting until it develops into osteoporosis. This could be half your female students over 50.

The starkest fact is that fractures after the age of 65 are associated with higher risks of mortality (Negrete-Corona et al, 2014). This is more the case for people in their 80s and 90s and you may not have many in your classes in that age group, but nonetheless it is significant and important.

It's important to remember that bones are not just structural; they are the storehouse of minerals that affect our entire system, from muscles to neurological impulses. There is also a hormone-like secretion from the bones, osteocalcin, which has been linked to improved insulin function and memory, among other things. So looking after bones is beneficial not just for the bones themselves.

Sarcopenia (muscle loss) is a condition seen most obviously in later life, but reduction in muscle mass starts earlier. Keeping an eye on muscle mass and strength is therefore essential too. All our work for bones is intertwined with supporting our muscles; the two go hand in hand. Any contraction of muscle will stimulate the periosteum (fascia around the bone), which in turn stimulates the genesis of bone tissue.

It is my conviction that if we are working with women we are doing them a disservice if we don't focus some of our offerings on bone strength and health, and protecting them from injury due to inappropriate asana, forceful adjustments, or falls. **Care of osteoporosis and osteopenia in yoga classes should not be thought of as a niche area.**

Can yoga help?

There is not enough rigorous and repeated evidence to definitively support the use of yoga to prevent or reverse osteoporosis. In my Yoga for Bone Health trainings I discuss why some research that may have lead you to believe otherwise is not robust, and what other avenues we can prioritize to support bones. However, a meta-analysis into the effects of Pilates and yoga on bone density found that these interventions resulted not in increased bone mass, but in a *maintenance* of bone in postmenopausal women. At a time when we would expect to see bone loss, this is encouraging. Note: better results were evident from Pilates than from yoga (Fernández-Rodríguez et al, 2021).

For the moment, the most robust research would lead us to be confident in saying that improving bone mass in postmenopause seems to be most reliably achieved by lifting heavy weight, multiple times per week, at an intensity of 80-85% of full effort (Watson et al, 2017). These are weights considerably greater than any you would be qualified or wise to include in your teaching and so would be better left to the gym.

In the general population, we also know that jumping, hopping, skipping, running, and dancing are beneficial (though advised against for people with fragility fractures). But remember, the effect of muscular action on bone growth is site-specific. This means that running and jumping will only positively affect the bones up as far as the lower one or two vertebrae, but not the rest of the spine—or the wrists, for instance.

How yoga can help

What I've just written may make you wonder what value you can possibly have for your clients with BMD loss. Wonder not! You have an excellent resource for this cohort. Bone health is not just about density, and yoga can help us to:

- develop all-over body conditioning that may make lifting weights and other forms of exercise safer (with "good form")
- increase muscular strength to aid stability and decrease fracture risk
- avoid falls through its balance challenges and proprioception stimulus
- feel more confident moving our body.

And you, as teachers, can help women after a diagnosis of osteopenia to feel confident as you expertly help them re-find movement at a time when they may feel unsure about what is safe anymore.

As a long-term yoga practitioner with osteoporosis, I know yoga doesn't guarantee everything. I also know the dismay as I stepped back on the mat wondering if yoga still had a safe place in my life. When I posted about vertebral compression fractures in yoga students, one reaction which lit a fire in me to figure this out for myself and my students was "these people would be better off not at yoga but going weight-lifting". Now, that's a valid statement. Weights are indeed the most reliably effective way to build bone, and some asana are unsafe for those with low BMD. But I thought to myself: How would it feel as a lover of yoga to be told by your teacher, "My classes are no longer relevant for you"? I believe if we learn enough we can keep our classes relevant and safe for all.

Protection first

Yoga can injure, of course. It can be tricky to know whether some injuries are a result of yoga, especially in the case of VCFs which can occur slowly over time. Though limited in that regard, one study found that "increased torsional and compressive mechanical loading pressures occurring during yoga SFE [spinal flexion exercises] resulted in de novo VCF [vertebral compression fractures]" (Sfeir et al, 2018). This was not a huge study, but I would not be happy to be the teacher that led even one person to a vertebral compression fracture or any other fracture.

The study concluded that "the appropriate selection of patients likely to benefit from yoga must be a cornerstone of fracture prevention." I would say that, rather than "selecting" patients (i.e., only those not at risk) and excluding those with osteopenia and osteoporosis, we should aim to make yoga safer for all.

- Teach balance and strength to maintain good posture and to avoid falls.
- Keep any students with osteopenia or osteoporosis whom you feel are at risk of falling near a wall during balance postures. (Sometimes, so as not to expose people who don't want to consider their vulnerability, I bring the whole class to the wall and then say they can use it or not as they see fit.)
- Avoid deep forward folds except with neutral spine. Never suggest pulling on toes to go further, and avoid levering or pushing into flexion.
- Offer back-strengthening exercises, because strong back muscles can reduce the risk of VCFs (Sinaki et al, 2002).
- Be cautious with hands-on adjustments and avoid pulling or pushing your student into any pose.
- Avoid end-of-range or twists of the spine, especially if there is a flexion included (whether intentional or unintentional).
- Avoid the student using the arms to lever into twists (especially avoid bound twists).

Adjusting some common postures for safety

When you approach postures or practices that have risks for osteoporosis, please consider including your students via variations rather than simply saying, "Don't do this if you have osteoporosis." For instance:

Child's pose

1) Avoid the flexion shown.

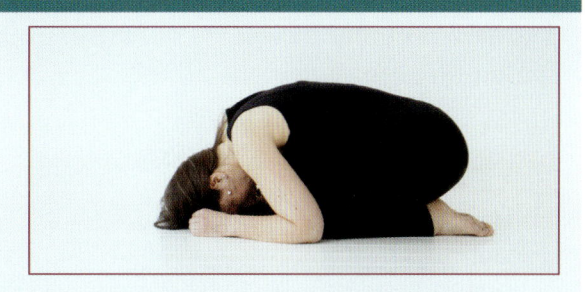

2) Maintain neutral spine throughout. This is done by allowing wider knees so the trunk can lower between the thighs rather than curving over them, extending the front body, and supporting the head on a block. This may be tricky for someone with hips or knees that are challenged by this considerable flexion.

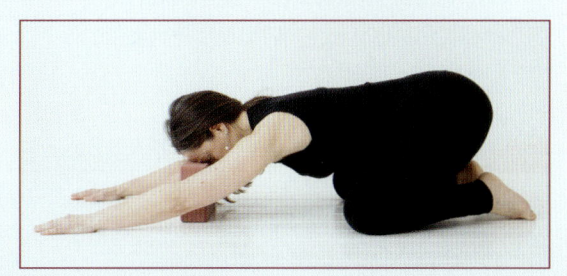

Cat/cow

1) Avoid excess flexion in cat, as seen on the left, but don't entirely avoid this movement, as it is still important to maintain some mobility. We are not aiming to stop movement, but to modulate it.

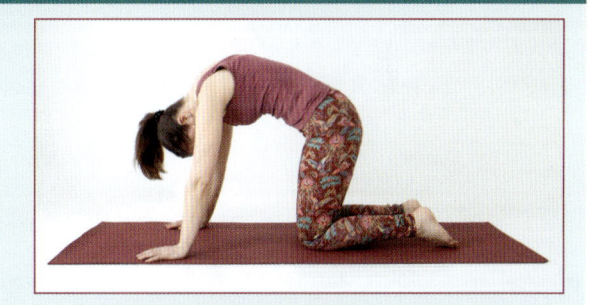

2) Allow the flexion to be controlled and muscular rather than pushing and reaching for an end-point in the shapes. Think of allowing a small amount of flexion coming from the tail tucking a little, and from abdominal effort. Avoid pushing down with the hands and arms.

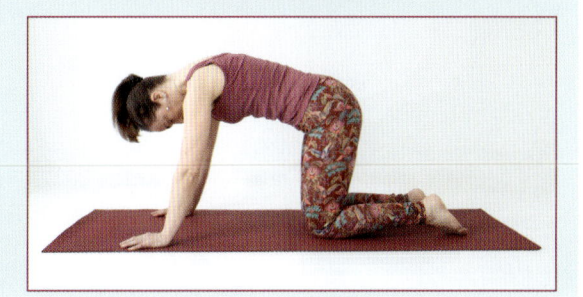

Safer twisting

The postures in the images are safer than, for example, half-lord of the fishes.

Twisting that involves the lumbar region may be more risky as it is not built for twisting, whereas the thoracic spine and neck are more accustomed to this motion.

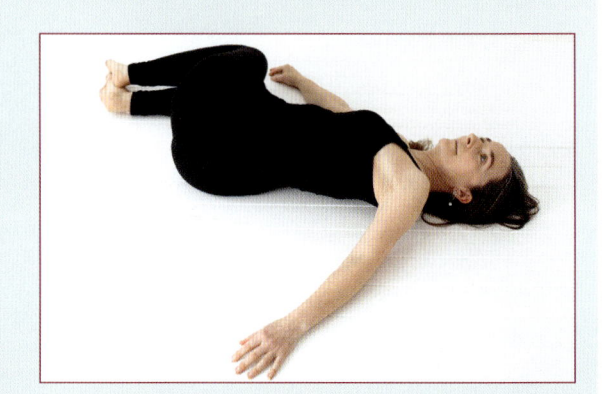

1) So keeping the pelvis neutral by stacking the top and bottom hips vertically, and aiming to twist more from the ribcage, without leverage, would be a little safer.

2) The hand resting on the shoulder, with a block to land on, may prevent over-twisting, and is especially useful for students who, when twisting, have difficulty easing the shoulder or arm to the floor. When the arm is elevated there can be a temptation to push it to the floor and pull the upper body over into more of a twist than is optimal for that person.

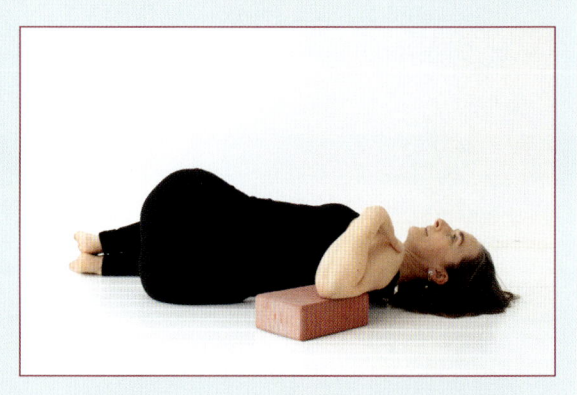

Downward-facing dog

This may seem safe as we are aiming for neutral spine, but when the focus is on straight legs and heels down, some spines will move into flexion where hamstrings are tight. So teach it with the knees bent, or start teaching it with hands on the wall (a standing dog) until a student has mastered neutral spine.

Triangle

As shown in the asana section about this posture, this can all too easily include both spinal flexion and twist at the same time. Consider teaching it in the way described in Chapter 2.

> ### Half-wheel
> If we aim for a big lift of the chest and don't adapt the neck angle, this is contraindicated. For instance, a lower lift into half-wheel will still create spinal and hip flexor extension. If we cue to stop with a straight line between the knees and throat, rather than an upward-curving bridge, instruct not to push the weight up to the shoulders and head, and cue to lift the chin away from the chest to encourage space between the back of the neck and the floor, we will avoid much of the extreme positioning and reduce the load placed on the vertebrae of the neck. Personally, I tend to avoid cueing the chin to the chest in any population anyway, to avoid neck strain.

Some common postures to avoid

Shoulder stand and **headstand** are contraindicated because of the load created in the cervical and thoracic spine, especially in the extreme neck position of shoulder stand.

Plough also creates considerable pressure on the neck and the whole spine because there is deep flexion throughout, but also because of the weight of the legs.

Bound twists like half-lord of the fishes and twisted side angle are unsafe for osteoporotic spines, as they involve twisting under pressure, and for many there will also be some spinal flexion.

While spinal extension is not contraindicated, **extreme backbends** are best avoided. Extension risks seem to be lower than in forward folding.

Ballistic stretch, like bouncing up and down to reach the toes, or passive stretch (using a strap or holding your toe to go further) in any direction would be riskier than keeping within active range of motion.

Needless to say, this is not an exhaustive list, and I hope that this whole section on bones will have given you sufficient information so that, as other postures come into your head or your teaching, you can determine yourself what might not be safe.

Getting to and from the floor

So if forward folds are tricky, then what happens to our lovely vinyasas and sun salutations? We adapt. And here's how!

116 YOGA FOR MENOPAUSE AND BEYOND

To get to all-fours and/or supine
This can be done also without a chair for those steady enough.

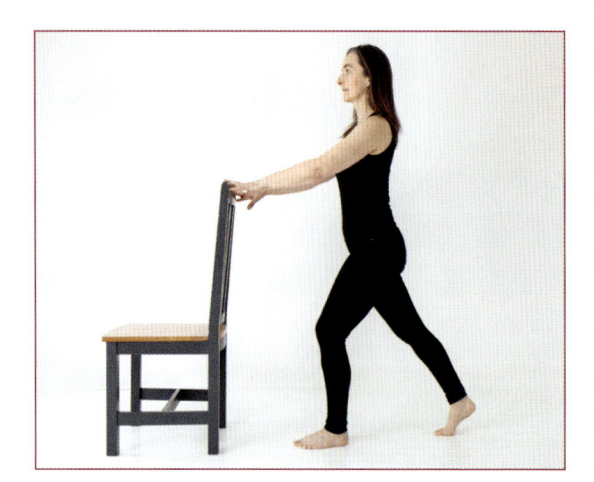

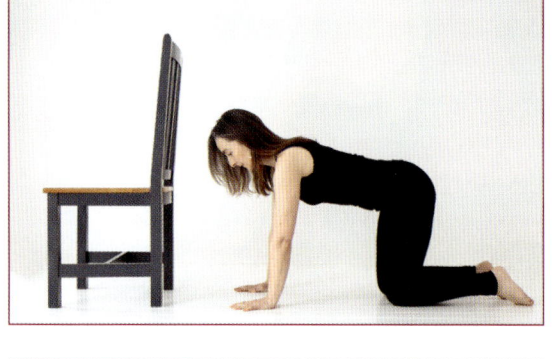

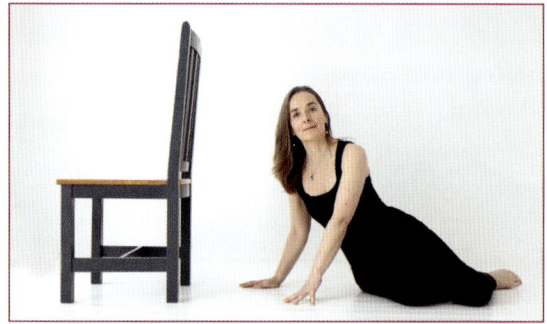

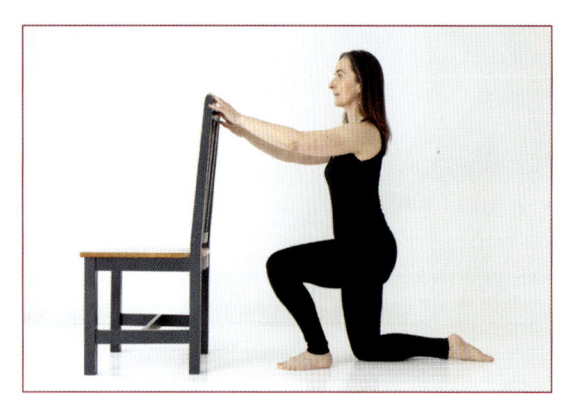

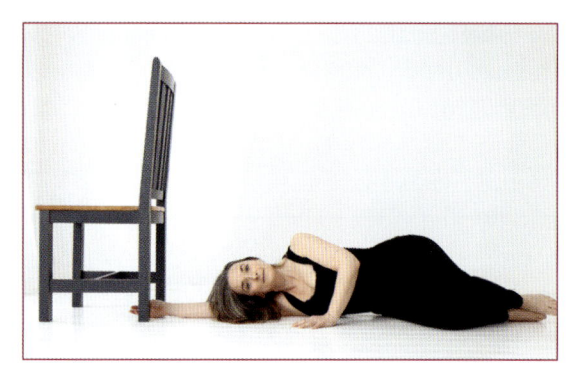

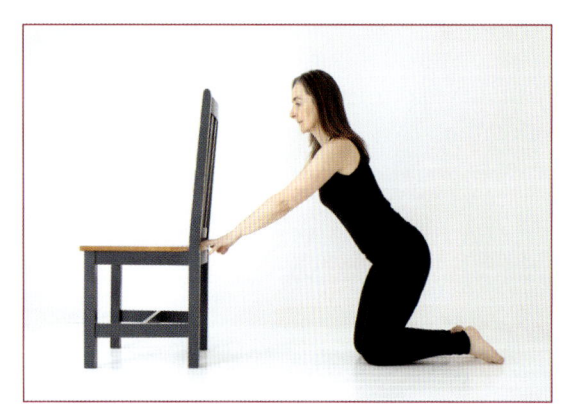

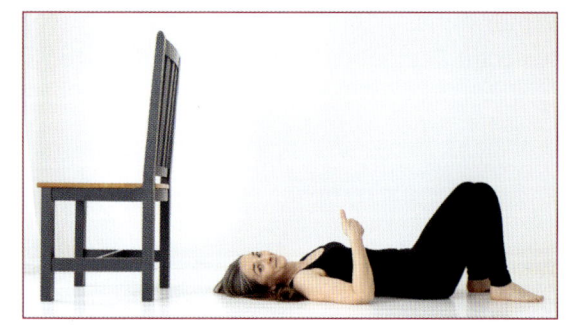

ENHANCING YOGA FOR MENOPAUSE HEALTH

An option for those who can squat

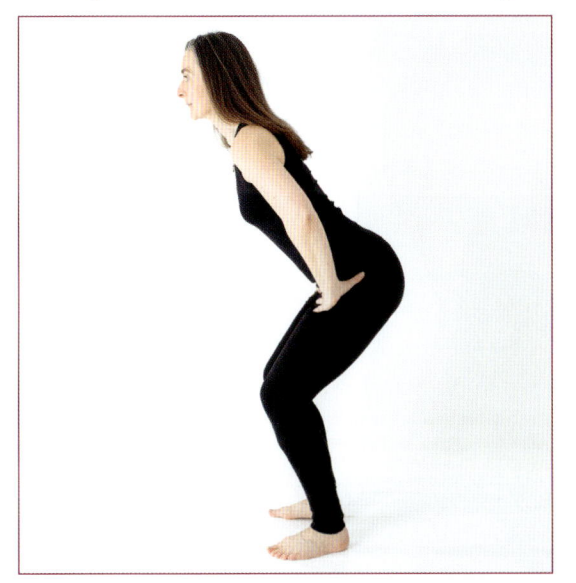

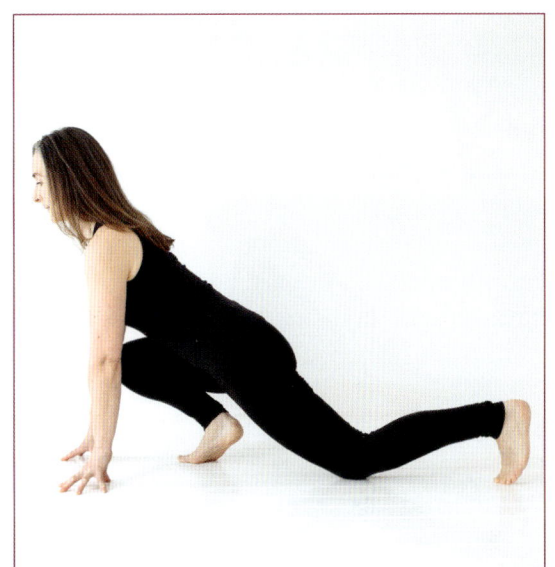

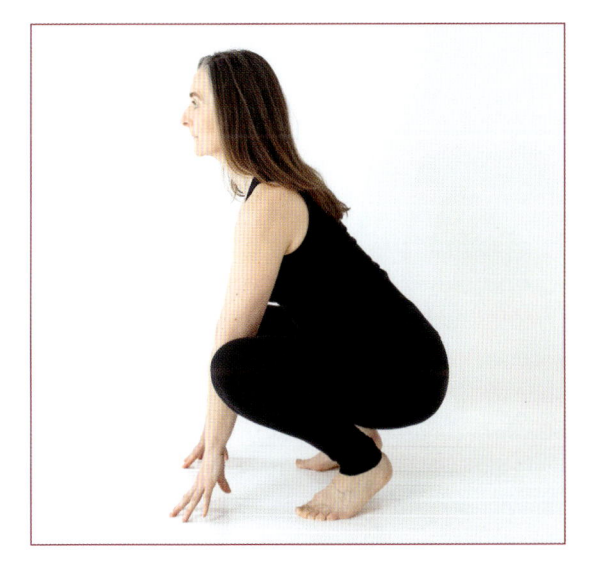

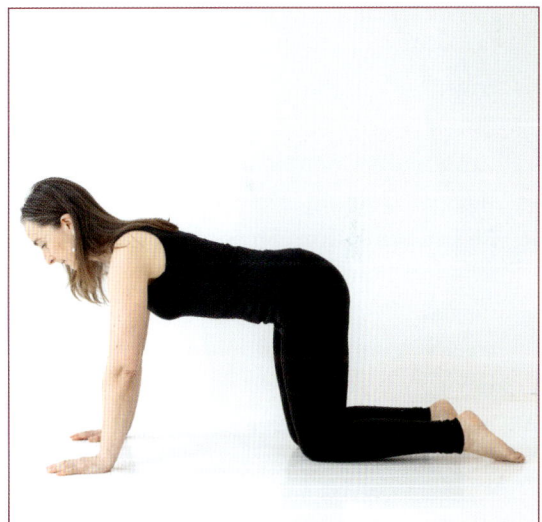

Yoga for bone health

Now that we have looked at prevention of fracture, or at least minimizing the risks, what follows are possibilities to enhance the level to which we can maintain bone health. Maintaining bone health is not just about increasing its density, but also about slowing its loss and protecting bones from compression and impact. So along with balance work there are other factors we should consider:

- **Strength.** If we want to target musculoskeletal strength more robustly we may need to include bands and weights, if you feel confident in doing so. This would be beneficial as a starting point for someone who is planning to incorporate strength training into their life, especially given that strength training can induce injury in sedentary people, so a build-up to heavier training is invaluable.
- **Stress reduction.** Stress negatively impacts bone and muscle mass because cortisol is catabolic (consuming tissue, essentially), so continue supporting the nervous system.
- **Mobility.** This a huge factor for independence and comfort in later life and for the avoidance of falls. So continue to support mobility, staying aware of contraindications and not offering gymnastic/contortionist-style asana.

Stimulating bone

We have been taught that to stimulate the laying down of new bone we need weight-bearing exercise (walking, running, dancing, weight-lifting), but there is research regarding the relationship of muscle and bone that also encourages the use of any muscular contraction:

> Several studies have indicated that higher muscle mass is closely related to increased BMD and reduced fracture risk in postmenopausal women… In addition, muscle and bone are simultaneously influenced by pathological states, such as glucocorticoid (cortisol for example) excess and vitamin D deficiency. These findings raise the possibility that there might be interactions between muscle and bone metabolism.
>
> Fractures that are covered with relatively intact muscle were found to improve more rapidly than fractures associated with more severe damage… These findings suggest that muscle tissues play important physiological and pathological roles through certain interactions between muscle tissues and bone metabolism. (Kaji, 2014)

So, though we know that lifting heavy weights is the gold standard for bone growth post-menopause, extrapolating from the above quote, we can hazard that any work to increase muscular mass has some positive effect on bone density, or at least, on reducing fracture risk and improving healing. By increasing isometric contraction, as detailed in the section on asana, we can add valuable muscular demand.

Weights and resistance bands

Though we cannot bring the kinds of heavy weights required to build bone into a yoga class, the addition of extra resistance with light weights and bands will support strength and stimulate bones more than bodyweight alone.

Weight-bearing exercise is more effective for people who have larger bodies and/or when carrying a rucksack, for instance. You could simply use wrist and ankle weights in your classes and not change a thing in your teaching. Or you can work with hand-held weights if you feel safe to do so.

Resistance bands are becoming more popular, and there is research that suggests that the results in muscular strengthening are comparable with the use of weights (Lopes et al, 2019).

Bands and hand weights are an increasingly common sight in yoga studios, and below I have included some ideas to help you add more positive stress on bones and muscles. I have not specified numbers of repetitions.

A general rule of thumb is that a person should lift a weight to the number of repetitions that does not involve exhaustion and maintains "good form" (she could do a few more with control and safety). However, heavy weights and lots of repetitions are not appropriate in a true yoga class.

If you are also a personal trainer you could do more, but at that point you might need to rename the class! If you don't feel comfortable adding non-yoga props, you could instead get creative with yoga belts and the weight of bolsters.

Exploring weights

A great addition to lunges is adding a lowering toward the floor and back up. From a high lunge, while still pressing the floor away from her, suggest that the student lowers the back knee almost to the floor, before coming back again. Go slow, perhaps in concert with the breath.

It's possible to make more demand on muscle and bone by the addition of weights while doing these movements. Your student could hold a bolster, or some books, or a couple of tins of beans!

- Slower movement is generally more muscularly demanding.
- However variety is something bones respond well to, so varying tempo can be valuable (for the brain too).
- Consider pressing the feet into the floor to come up.
- You can hold the weight statically, close to the body or overhead, or add arm movements like bicep and tricep curls, elevating and lowering the arms with each lowering and raising of the knee.
- The more/less you grip the weights, the more/less muscular engagement there will be.
- Engage mula bandha and a little uddiyana bandha or engage the PF and abdomen, as guided in p.144.

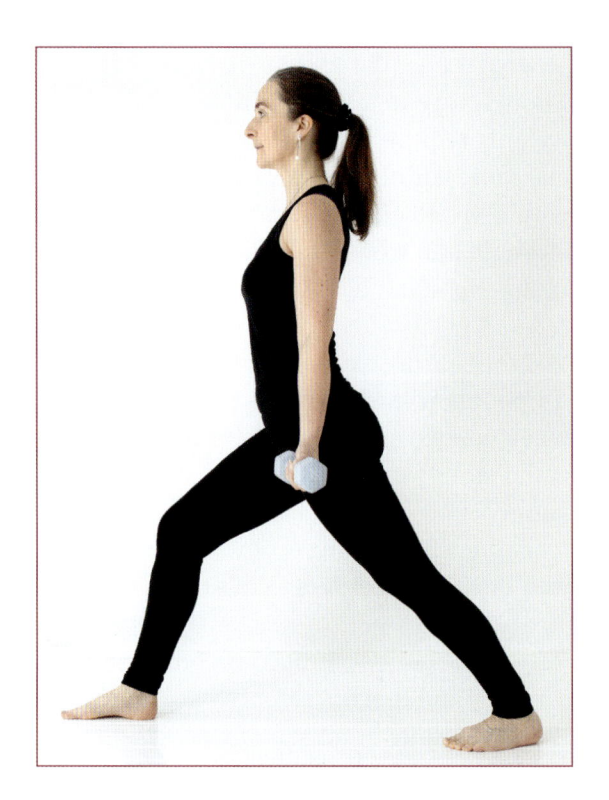

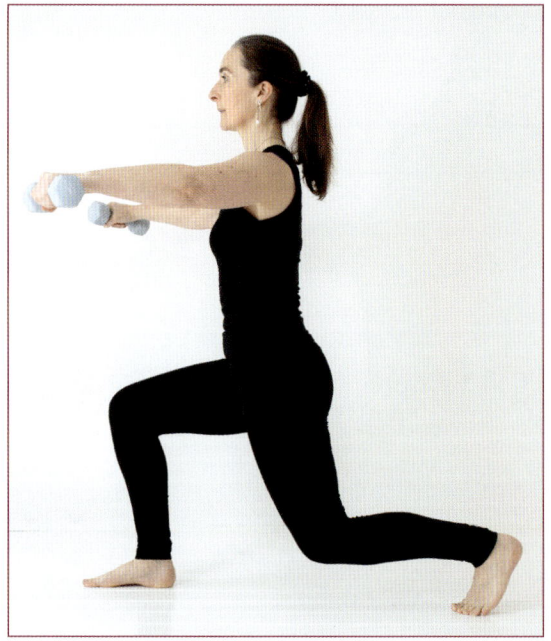

Simply holding weights as you move through some postures can be really effective as a reminder not to take postures too far, as the added weight makes the body a bit more chatty when it starts to feel over-challenged! I find holding weights is particularly effective for ensuring good spinal alignment and core engagement.

As well as adding strength control and postural awareness, arm movements mid-posture can also demand a more focused mind, especially if the arms are being asked to make asymmetrical movements.

The images below might give you some ideas.

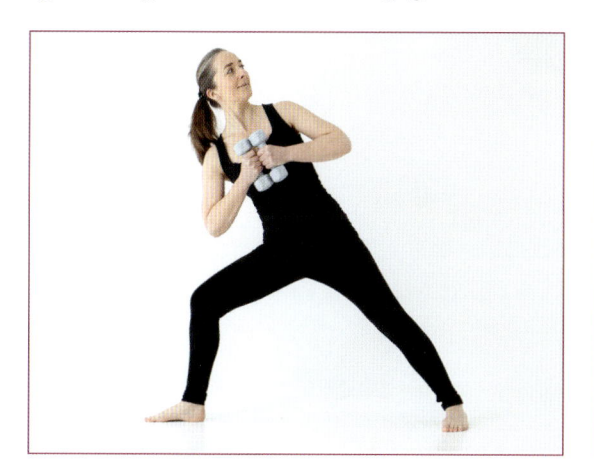

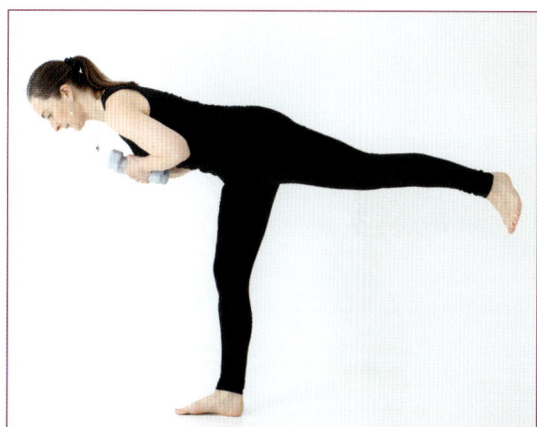

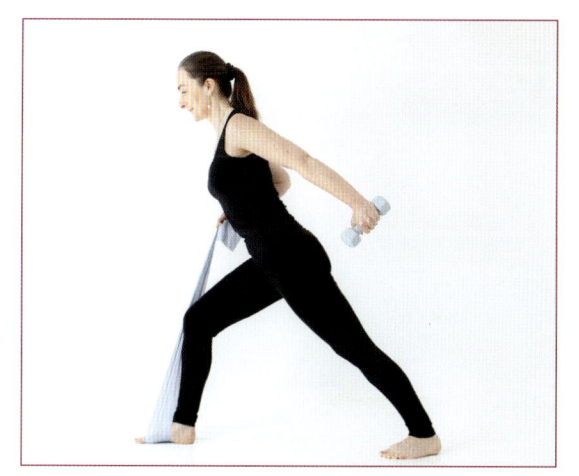

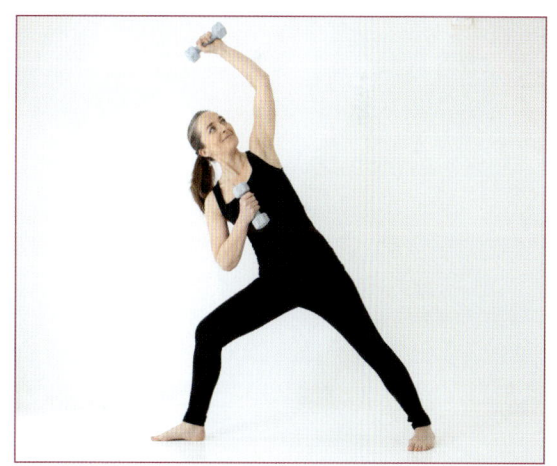

More weight drills

Pull-ups. These can be done in lunges, in warrior, with squats, or in mountain pose. Watch out for excess neck or shoulder tension.

Triceps curls. Can also be done on all-fours and in any standing or even many balancing postures. Look out for rounding of the spine.

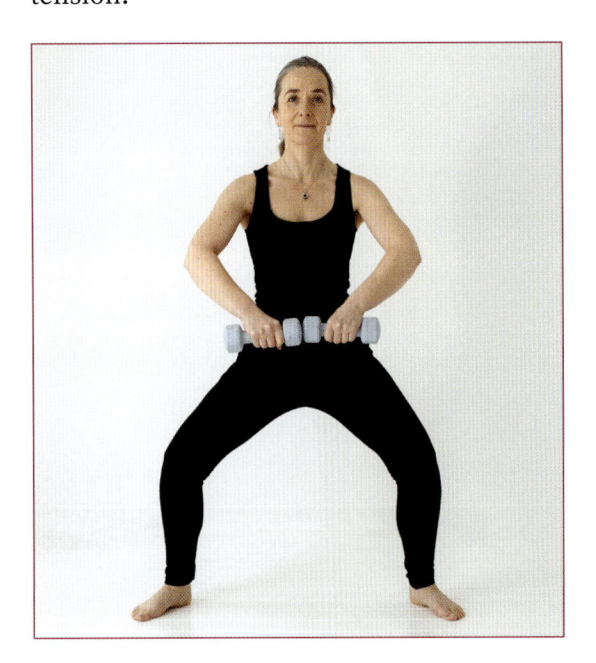

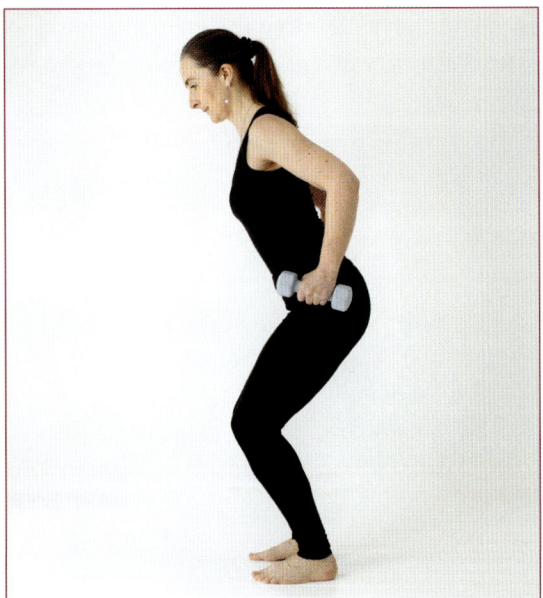

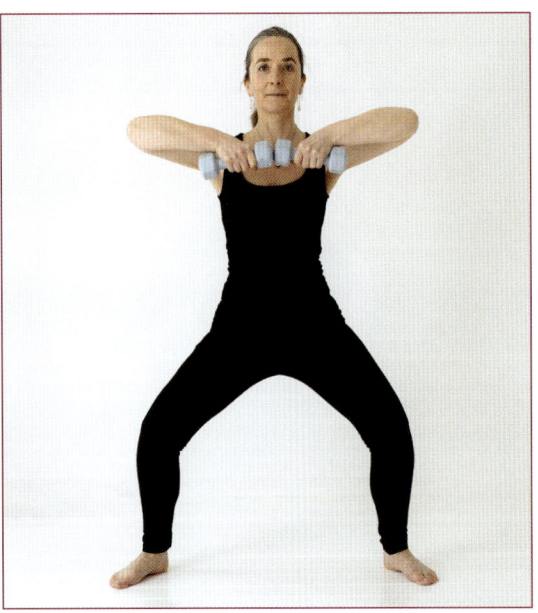

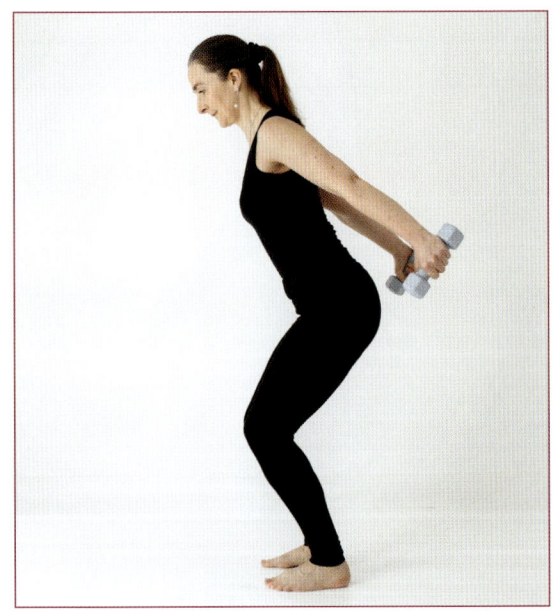

Lateral arm raises. Harder than they look: raise the arms less high, and keep a little bend in the elbow to avoid deltoid strain.

Why so much focus on the arms? Spinal osteogenesis is notoriously difficult to engender, partly because, as I said, the muscular stimulation of bone growth is site-specific. Working our arms works our back muscles. Stronger back muscles also help with posture, which helps prevent falls, and are associated with fewer VCFs.

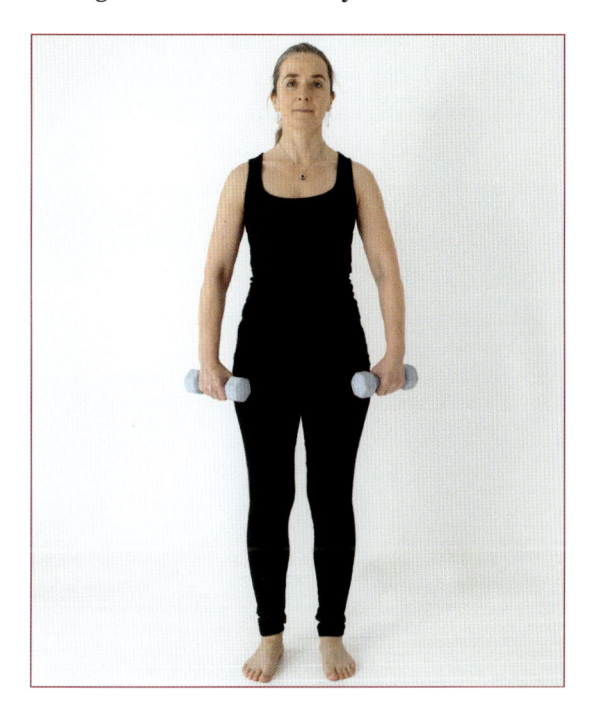

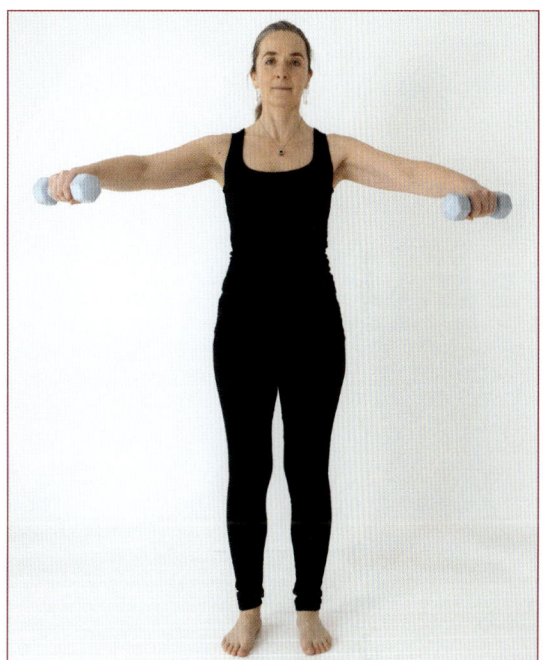

Resistance bands

In all the resistance band work, the aim is to maintain the band in an engaged rather than loose state, even when returning to the starting point of repetitious movements.

Warrior I

1) With bands around wrists, arms elevated, push arms gently outward against resistance. Soften shoulders and keep a slight bend in the elbows. Beware of using too strong a band, especially when arms are elevated.

2) Progress to lateral pull-downs as the elbows bend outward and the band journeys behind the head. Engage mula bandha and the core muscles. You can also do these movements seated on a chair or standing.

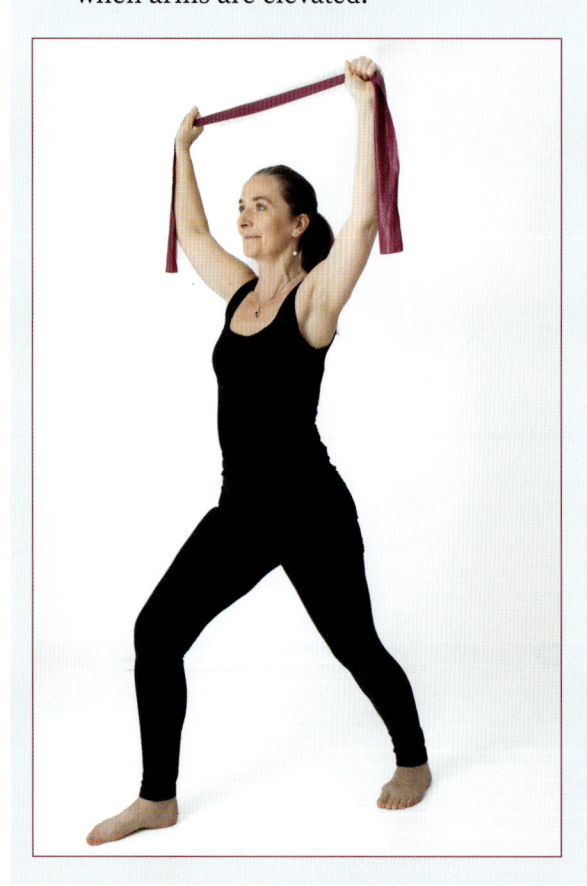

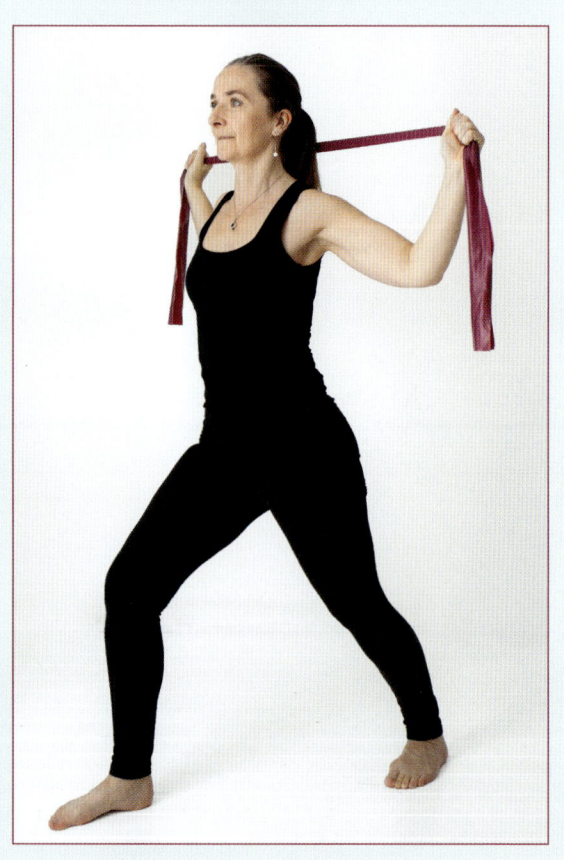

Downward dog

Place a circular band around one ankle and the opposite foot. Perform a single leg raise on the side where the band is on the foot. If you have a single long band, tie a small loop at one end for the foot and hold the other end with the same-side hand. Look out for anyone lifting the leg too high. Instead keep the pelvis level.

Swap sides. A couple of reps each side is tough enough!

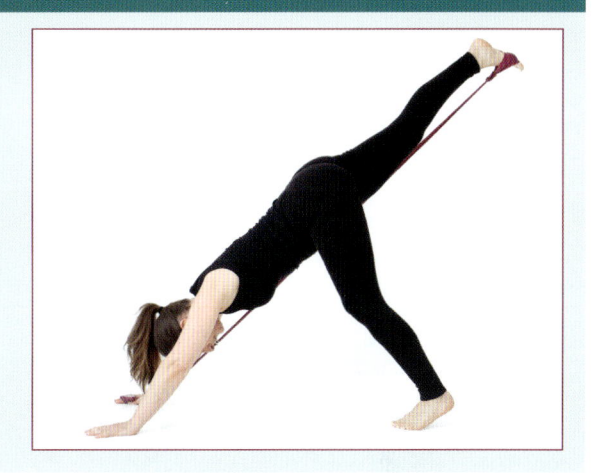

Locust pose

Lying on the belly with the band around the ankles, tone the bandhas, press the pubic bone into the mat, lift legs and move feet apart and together. Small movements are plenty. Keep the legs low. This is strong and may be too much for some lower back issues. Be cautious.

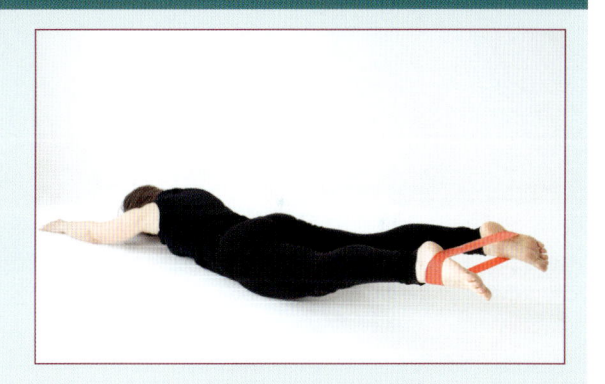

For the core

1) Lie semi-supine. Engage mula bandha and the lower abdomen, both of which are more activated on the exhale. Raise your legs with thighs at right angles to your body. Place the bands around the balls of your feet only, or thighs also. Slowly extend alternate legs at an angle of about 30–45 degrees to the floor.
2) Add light weights for extra complexity and eustress.

I use principles of Pilates to enhance what yoga offers. I didn't really understand the core, and other muscles of the trunk that can add to strength, stability and proprioception until I trained in Pilates. Even if you never intend to teach it, it is a training you may consider.

Lots more band work can be added in warrior and other poses. There are trainings in use of resistance bands in yoga out there if you are interested in specializing.

Please remember that what I have offered you here are only a few examples of a vast array of things you can do in a vast array of positions.

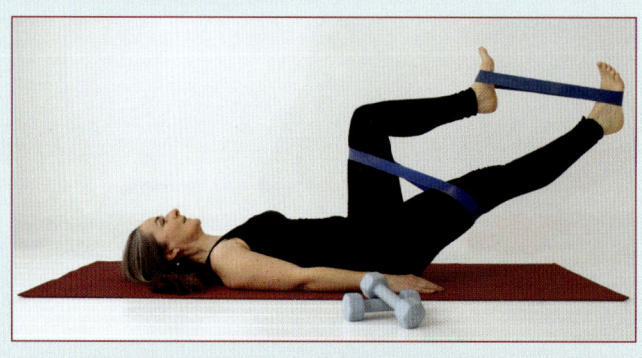

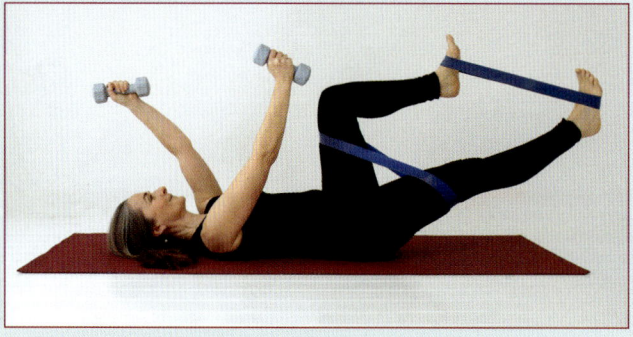

Jumping

Things like running and downhill walking stimulate the bones because of the percussive action. The effects of jumping and hopping have also been seen to be beneficial to bones. One of the warm-ups my first teacher taught me was trotting up and down the length of our mats. You can easily add such trotting or jumping on the spot to a standing warm-up. You may need to teach just heel-taps (only the heels leave the floor) for anyone concerned about falling or at high risk of fracture, and/or ask students to perform it while holding a wall, just as you would with balancing postures. Most women who are not frail should be okay to do little jumps on an even surface.

While performing, say, 50 little jumps, focusing on creating tangible, even audible percussion, you could point out how easy it would be for them to add these into their lives.

Posture and balance

The prevention of fractures owing to falls, and avoiding the compression of vertebrae that can occur from an increased kyphosis, may be more achievable by working on balance, back strength, and posture than by lifting heavy weights two to three times a week forever.

Please see the balance challenges that I have included in the section in Chapter 4 b) on p.137 and consider them part of your protection of students with osteopenia and osteoporosis. There are techniques there that address posture too. Working on foot mobility, strength, and awareness is valuable for functional balance (i.e., while performing everyday tasks like walking). Yoga in general is already good for all these areas, but the techniques added in this book truly enhance the resources of this rich tradition.

Support outside yoga—nutrition

You can exercise like a pro weightlifter and athlete, but if you don't eat enough, there are insufficient resources to create bone mineral density. Some basic guidelines:

- Don't scrimp on protein. Have some at every meal, for bone and muscle health.
- Collagen is the structure of all our tissues, including bones, and supplementing seems to be getting good results for joints in studies (Clark et al, 2008; García-Coronado et al, 2019).
- Collagen is naturally available by consuming fish with bones, and the skin and connective tissue of animals.
- Protein will help us make collagen. Vitamin C helps us use it.
- Calcium is found in: dairy, soy, cashews, almonds, green leafy veg, sesame seeds, beans, lentils, dried fruit, and in fish when bones are eaten.
- Magnesium and other minerals are important too. Available in all the above, and in all nuts, seeds (especially pumpkin), seaweed, molasses, wholegrains, bananas.
- When consuming calcium-rich foods, frequent small amounts spread over the day are best.
- Vitamin K is important, and can be found in: chicken, oily fish, egg yolk, liver. K2 may be more important and is found in fermented food.
- Vitamin D is essential for bone health and should be supplemented in winter months.
- Calcium supplements should only be used under medical or qualified nutritional advice for over-50s because of risks to heart health.
- Taking a calcium supplement is safer with D and K2 (ideally from a food source rather than a supplement) at the same time.
- Hydration is immensely important, supporting, among other things, the movement of minerals to the bones.

B) BRAIN

The changing biology

A survey by dementiastatistics.org found that Alzheimer's has become the most feared disease of later life. You read in Chapter 1 about some of the effects reproductive aging has on the brain. There is a huge amount of discussion in the media at the time of writing this book about changes to the brain wrought by menopause, and conflicting evidence as to whether MHT might accelerate, slow, or make no difference to the development of Alzheimer's disease. Women in menopause are facing a lot of confusion and fear about their brain and how to protect it.

Some evidence shows that the brain changes associated with Alzheimer's disease begin in our 20s and 30s, long before perimenopause, which puts a bit of perspective on the current narrative that it's perimenopause that puts us at risk. What is the truth of it? I don't claim to know the definitive answer. What is certainly true is that women notice brain-related symptoms of menopause. So maybe it doesn't matter what the cause is, because looking after our brain is always worthwhile.

In their research on the female brain in menopause, Lisa Mosconi and her team found:

> substantial differences in brain structure, connectivity, and energy metabolism across MT stages ... These effects involved brain regions subserving higher-order cognitive processes and were specific to menopausal endocrine aging rather than chronological aging, as determined by comparison to age-matched males.

And:

> Brain **biomarkers** largely **stabilized** post-menopause, and **gray matter volume** (GMV) **recovered** in key brain regions for cognitive aging. Notably, GMV recovery and in vivo brain mitochondria ATP production correlated with preservation of cognitive performance post-menopause, suggesting **adaptive compensatory processes.** (Mosconi et al, 2021; my bold)

The brain in menopause shows some scary changes. But encouragingly, it also shows *recoverability*.

The brain is one of the least understood and most complex systems known to humanity, but it also seems to be one of the most adaptable: Neurons that have died can revive, and new neurons and new neural connections can be made. This neuroplasticity is why people who have lost certain areas of capability after strokes can learn these things again, sometimes using different brain regions.

We can assume that every brain that arrives to us as teachers needs to be fed. The brain needs fuel and activation to keep vital. It can't store energy in the same way muscles can store fat to use for energy in times of low nourishment, so it needs adequate, regular nutritional intake to keep fueled. But just like muscles, it will atrophy if it is unused and unchallenged.

We see fewer incidents of symptomatic Alzheimer's disease in those who are learning, have a depth of language and ideas, who learn new physical things, who have spiritual connection, and who have purpose in life. This may be why we have evidence of brains with the physiological changes of Alzheimer's disease where the individual is/was symptom-free. I highly recommend you read the Nun Study (Iacono et al, 2009), or at least an article on it, especially if you find this section alarming. Alzheimer's disease has a good profile in terms of our ability to protect ourselves through lifestyle measures.

A spiritual element

Spiritual "fitness" is spoken of as another indicator of lower risk of cognitive decline. In an article in Alzheimersprevention.org, spiritual fitness is described thus, regardless of religion if any:

- Socialization or being with like-minded people
- Acceptance and forgiveness of yourself and others
- Patience and allowing yourself to be in the moment
- Compassion and empathy toward yourself and others
- Purpose or meaning in life via self-discovery and building your legacy.

Yoga, right?!

But can we help more? I think so.

How yoga can help

Because brains are so responsive to everything we do, there are many ways we can support them. To consider how we can help through yoga, let's first see what's recommended in the mainstream:

- **Physical exercise**
- **Mental exercise, especially increase novelty (new learning)**
- **Staying social**
- **Prioritizing sleep improvement**
- **Regulating stress**
- **Treating or avoiding high blood pressure (BP)**
- **Treating and aiming to avoid unstable blood sugar to reduce diabetes risk**
- **Treating depression**
- **Aiming to maintain a sense of purpose**
- Stopping smoking
- Reducing alcohol consumption
- Treating hearing loss (hearing aids)
- Eating lots of fruit, vegetables, protein, and good fats.

You can see that yoga targets the areas in bold already, so even without the enhancements below, your classes are already helping.

More specifically, there is some encouraging clinical testing that shows that Kirtan Kriya meditation, from the Kundalini yoga (KY) practice, can help with cognitive function and memory. It also helped stimulate the sensory-motor cortex.

> *Kirtan Kriya meditation has been shown to mitigate the deleterious effects of chronic stress on cognition, reverse memory loss, and create psychological and spiritual wellbeing, which may reduce multiple drivers of Alzheimer's disease risk.* (Khalsa & Newberg, 2021)

> *Both KY and MET [memory enhancement training] groups showed significant improvement in memory; however, only KY showed significant improvement in executive functioning. Only the KY group showed significant improvement in depressive symptoms and resilience.* (Eyre et al, 2017)

My sense is that this is effective because singing, humming, and chanting stimulate the vagus nerve, and coordinating new movements in rhythm and with sounds stimulates the brain. You will easily find instruction in this practice on YouTube or similar.

The vagus nerve

I believe that yoga's chief benefit for brain health is its clear support of the nervous system—in particular, the vagus nerve (VN). Because some yoga practices are very repetitious, once learnt, they may not be as beneficial for the stimulus of new neurological growth as they were when the practitioner was learning them. That's why I am offering you some of the additional brain stimulus techniques that follow.

But yoga continues to support the brain, which always wants to know it is safe, through calming the nervous system, in part via practices known to support the VN. So below I offer you an overview of this important part of our nervous system, as it too will support brain health.

The vagus nerve (thus called in reference to its "vagrant" nature, wandering widely as it does) runs from the brain stem to the viscera and back again, and affects all our organs. It is part of the autonomic nervous system, of which the parasympathetic nervous system (PSNS) and the sympathetic nervous system (SNS) are constituents.[2] In fact, "autonomic" is a slight misnomer, as it implies that we have no control over which part of our nervous system is activated at any one time, whereas we now know that we can encourage PSNS dominance. The PSNS is the arm of the nervous system that helps us to rest, relax, and repair, and can only activate when we feel safe; the SNS helps us escape from threat and get things done, and is activated when we feel overwhelmed as well as if there is a tiger chasing us.

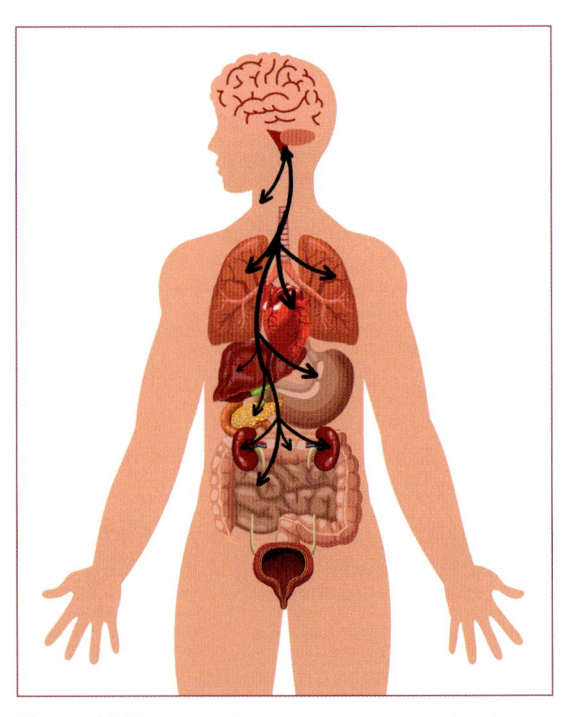

Figure 4.1 *The complex vagus nerve put simply!*

---

[2] *Though these are more properly termed the parasympathetic and sympathetic arms of the autonomic nervous system, in this book I will use the more common terms, PSNS and SNS, as shorthand.*

The vagus nerve (or actually, these nerves, because there are two) is known to be responsible for the stimulation of the PSNS, and its tone—or lack thereof—is a significant factor in our ability to deactivate the SNS when it has done its job. Put simply: the better your vagal tone, the easier it is for you to relax.

Low vagal tone is not just about being unable to come into rest-and-restore mode. It is associated with a number of issues. Those which are of particular interest to us as we support the symptoms of menopause would be: depression, chronic fatigue, diabetes, digestive issues, cardiovascular conditions, inflammatory conditions, and cognitive impairment.

High vagal tone improves blood sugar regulation, cardiovascular health, blood pressure, digestion, and migraines. It is associated with better mood, less anxiety, and more stress resilience.

There is debate in the medical and scientific communities as to how to test for vagal tone. The most common way has been to measure heart rate between the inhalation and the exhalation, and the greater the variability, the greater the tone. Another layman's route has been to determine heart rate variability under different circumstances, i.e., from rest to exertion and back again. If the heart rate variability is high, this has been used as a marker to indicate high vagal tone.

Really it doesn't matter, as you will not be testing, only supporting. As yoga teachers, diagnosis is not our job. But we can certainly use many techniques from yoga to stimulate the VN, and many of these are well within the realm of our expertise. Central to the advice I give is about how women can find ways to increase stress positively and then return to PSNS activation, and become adept at inducing both responses because they choose to. In class, that looks like little bursts of activity creating demand, either on muscle or mind, followed by mini-rests and actions supportive of the VN.

You will see that many interventions recommended in this book for symptoms and long-term health are based on stimulating the PSNS, which is controlled by the vagus nerve.

How yoga supports the VN

First let's congratulate ourselves for bringing to our students a tradition that has clinically proven benefits for the nervous system. There are not many areas where yoga has such definitive and repeatable outcomes as in the area of stress.

Yoga has been demonstrated to:

- Decrease perceived stress (Shohani et al, 2018)
- Reduce SNS dominance (Shobana et al, 2022)
- Increase PSNS dominance (Shobana et al, 2022)
- Decrease cortisol (Thirthalli et al, 2013)
- Possibly increase GABA, a calming neurotransmitter (Streeter et al, 2010)
- Increase dopamine (Kjaer et al, 2002).

These effects are seen particularly in regular practitioners; it may take a while for beginners to experience them.

In addition, vagal tone benefits from:

- Exercise (we enjoy) that varies heart rate
- Slow diaphragmatic breathing
- Stimulation of the vocal folds and throat (speaking, yawning, singing, laughing, humming, and ujjayi breathing)
- Social engagement
- Massage (even self-massage)
- Meditation, including metta and karuna, which increases goodwill toward others, improving the ability to socially engage and bond.

Outside yoga, cold water exposure, probiotics and the consumption of foods rich in omega-3s are a few other things for which research has been done or is ongoing that indicate benefits for VN tone.

We see that the better the vagal tone, the better our ability to engage in the practices which improve tone—and so on, in a positive cycle. We are essentially endeavoring to improve a woman's ability to return to parasympathetic predominance after the sympathetic arousal caused by a stressful circumstance has passed.

Stimulating the brain

Let's get back to the brain itself. Here I offer you a little insight into what makes it tick. The brain's main concern at all times is "Can I trust you?" It relies on our neurotransmitter signals to help it see and feel safe. If the input is clear and reliable, and not putting our organism in danger, the brain will trust us and be happy enough to allow PSNS activity. This can give us more freedom and comfort because when we are in SNS arousal, the brakes are on; muscles are contracted ready for action. In PSNS arousal, we are less flexed and more mobile.

Interestingly, giving the brain complex challenges like the hand exercise on p.136 can also increase flexibility. This may be because the brain feels safe while you are challenging it, or because it is so complex as to be meditative. (I challenge you to be able to think of anything other than the exercise while doing it. You will truly be one-pointed in the mind!) The brain likes to know that you/it are adaptable to a range of circumstances. Teaching it new things assists it to be adaptable.

So we seek to help it trust us by not putting our tissues in danger, and by giving it enough fuel and activation so it knows it is ready for anything.

Look at figure 4.2, a rough map of the brain: the four areas outlined in white indicate the approximate location of the more primitive parts of the brain that reside between the two outer halves. We will be looking into a few of these regions in a moment.

But first, knowing what you now know, consider which brain regions you would want to stimulate most. Of course, as I have said, stimulating any region will have a

ENHANCING YOGA FOR MENOPAUSE HEALTH   133

Frontal Lobe
Working memory, anxiety, sharpness of intellect, movement, concentration, personality, depression

Sensory Motor Cortex
Voluntary muscular control, skin sensations

Parietal Lobe
Sensations, language, perception, body awareness, attention

Thalamus
Sleep, consciousness, alertness

Occipital Lobe
Vision, perception

Temporal Lobe
Hearing, language, memory

Cerebellum
Balance, posture, coordination

Hypothalamus
Temperature regulation, sleep, hunger, energy

Vestibular System
Balance, dizziness

Limbic Cortex
Made up of thalamus, hypothalamus, amygdala, hippocampus, and more. Memory, information processing, emotion, motivation

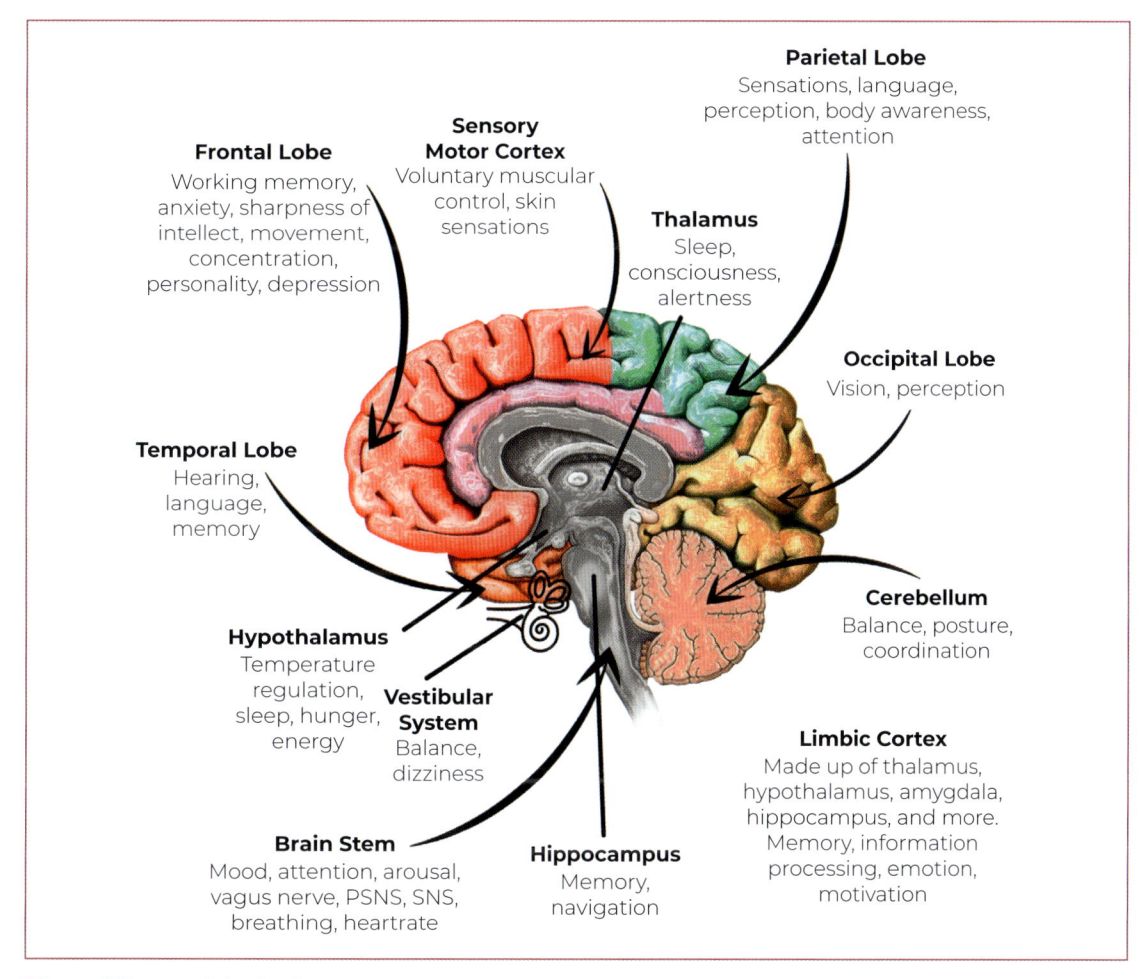

Brain Stem
Mood, attention, arousal, vagus nerve, PSNS, SNS, breathing, heartrate

Hippocampus
Memory, navigation

Figure 4.2 *Map of the brain*

positive effect for the whole brain so don't get too concerned with specific areas. But asking yourself that question will get your own cogs whirring and get you thinking laterally with the new information you have. This is a key to being a good teacher—joining the dots from what you have learned to what you can offer.

Given the main kinds of brain-related menopause symptoms, I tend to focus on the following areas:

1) **Frontal lobe:** Regulates emotions in interpersonal relationships and social situations, including emotions that are considered positive (happiness, gratitude, satisfaction) and negative (anger, jealousy, pain, sadness). It is also

involved in memory, impulse control, problem solving, and motor function. Damage to the neurons or tissue of the frontal lobe can lead to personality changes, difficulty concentrating or planning, and impulsivity.

2) **Brain stem:** Connects the cerebrum and cerebellum to the spinal cord. It performs many automatic functions such as regulating breathing, heart rate, body temperature, wake and sleep cycles, digestion, sneezing, coughing, vomiting, and swallowing. The vagus nerve connects it to the spine. It is the area responsible for PSNS and SNS balance.

3) **Cerebellum:** Adjusts posture to maintain balance. Input is from vestibular receptors and proprioceptors, then it decodes instructions going to motor neurons to compensate for shifts in body position or changes in load upon muscles. Essentially it simplifies input coming up the spine.

4) **Vestibular system:** Supports balance and awareness of positioning when we are moving. It works in collaboration with the visual system, including our eyes, their muscles and parts of the brain that create the experience of seeing. The cerebellum and vestibular systems are intimately connected, and the visual system intimately connected with the vestibular.

Before you read the next paragraph, pause and have a think about why I prioritize these areas. See if you notice how your growing awareness is changing or influencing the way you think about the body, the mind, and how yoga can support their changing needs in peri- and post-menopause.

Now I'll tell you why!

1) **Frontal lobe.** I think this one is pretty obvious. In perimenopause, relationships and social situations can feel very much more stressful, triggering, and unappealing than hitherto. Emotional regulation may seem harder, and concentration and memory are at a premium in perimenopause. Concentration and memory issues can continue after menopause, and many people find these tendencies very worrying.

2) **Brain stem.** This is, of course, all to do with helping to regulate the stress response so we feel better, sleep better, and can reduce risks of higher-than-optimal inflammation. Though there is very little to be done about frequency of hot flushes other than MHT/HRT, any reduction in stress has a positive impact on them, and on issues like palpitations, anxiety, and digestion.

3) **Cerebellum.** I include this region because I am passionate about helping women with osteoporosis avoid falls.

4) **Vestibular system.** Likewise, this system is central to balance during functional movement, and it's also fun and easy to challenge it.

Please note, if you or your student experience nausea or dizziness during any brain challenges, this is a sign that the nervous system is confused and overloaded, and is a stress too far. It can occur, for instance, when the visual and vestibular senses are sending contradictory information to the brain, as with car sickness when reading: the eyes think we're not moving, but the vestibular system senses we are. When we look out at the moving landscape, eventually the nausea fades.

In the case of nausea or dizziness, pull back.

Support outside yoga

In my yoga teacher training I teach a module I call Neuroanatomy and Brain-Food in Movement. Below are some snippets of the kinds of things you can add for brain food. It would not be appropriate or possible to teach some of the techniques in writing, so these are simply outlines of possibilities for you to research.

Please note: I am not suggesting that by adding these elements to your classes you will be ensuring that your students avoid Alzheimer's disease or other forms of dementia, but we know that challenging the brain is a positive move for long-term brain and cognitive health.

Brain snacks

I suggest you offer these brain snacks by saying they are a way to keep the brain lively and energized. Though you can share that movement novelty seems to be positive for brain health, remember that there are many reasons someone may develop these diseases. Neither you nor they can say that something they tried didn't work or that they failed to protect their brain by not doing x, y, or z enough or "properly."

Adding these and other fun challenges can increase activation and demand, helping the brain feel alert and capable, while building new neurological connections.

I have put in brackets after each one a number referring to the brain region mostly stimulated (as numbered above).

Cognitive load

Don't let your students auto-pilot their way through your class. Challenge them, and yourself, by not repeating the same old same old over and over.

- Teach a few variations of a movement, giving each a number and instructing their performance by saying the number instead of the action. For example, on all-fours instruct cat/cow, then child/kneeling plank, then table-top with extended arm and opposite leg, and give them numbers. Then, call out the numbers as the only instruction so they have to remember what action to perform. Speed up the changes between each movement to make it harder. (1)
- Offer saccades (detailed below) with contrary instruction (right for left, down for up, etc.). (1)
- Perform an asana with added eye practices. (1, 2, 4)
- Eyes-closed balance and/or movement. (2, 4)

Sequencing and stacking

Learning new sequences is a great brain challenge, and stacking further challenge on top can ensure that, when something becomes too easy, there is more positive stress available.

- Offer a new short sequence in each class that the student has to remember themselves and perform after a short time. (1)
- Offer non-dominant effort in control and strength (e.g., more balancing on non-dominant leg, asymmetrical movements, coordination challenges, lunging back and forth with the dominant foot staying in the center of the mat, and the non-dominant stepping to the top and back of the mat over and over). (2)
- Offer any posture with added complexity (as above but also add, for instance, tilting the head, eye movements as detailed below, speed changes students must follow of any rhythmical movements). (1, 2, 4)

Have fun adding the mind-bender in this image. Instructions are in Chapter 5 a) on p.165.

Memory has been seen to be better in people who are mixed-handed (Parker et al, 2017). Perhaps in the majority who aren't, training the non-dominant limb might help.

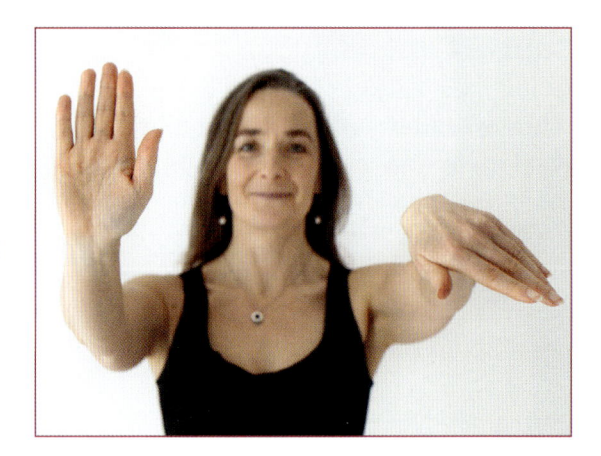

Vestibular system challenges

Of course, challenging the vestibular system should never go as far as inducing nausea, or falling. But stimulating it by taking the body off center, and adding chosen extra challenges like head or eye movements can help it to be more responsive to a range of tricky circumstances, helping to reduce the risk of falling. These challenges are thus good for the brain (challenging it) and for bone safety, within safe limits.

I call this the Titanic Tilt because it's like the way the body naturally responds to being on the deck of a ship on the sea.

1) Tilt over forward from the ankles until you are just about to fall. Stay a while before tilting back.
2) Make sure not to bend at the waist or hips or it's not a brain challenge!

It's a great start to a class, really helping with interoception as we feel neurology and muscle so clearly working to stabilize.

3 & 4) In any balancing (or even standing) pose, move the head to different orientations to add challenge. Begin with slow movements, then over the weeks, add challenge by

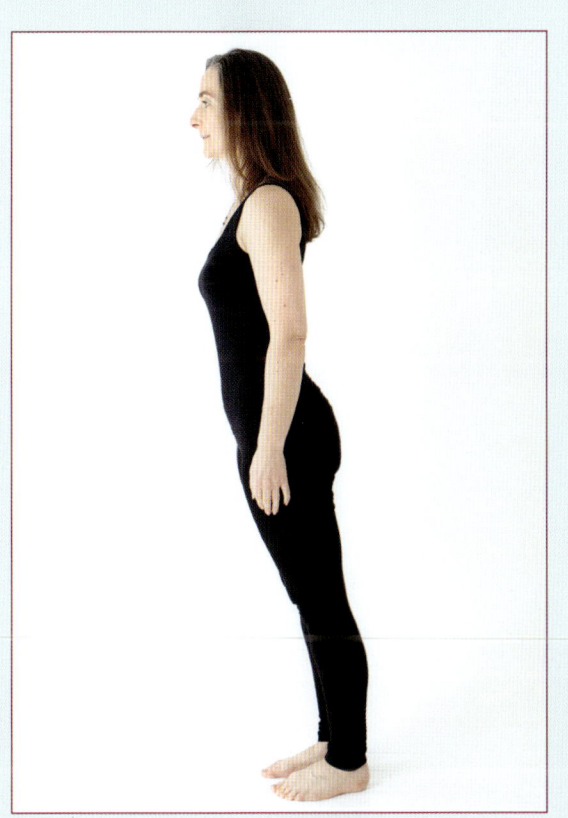

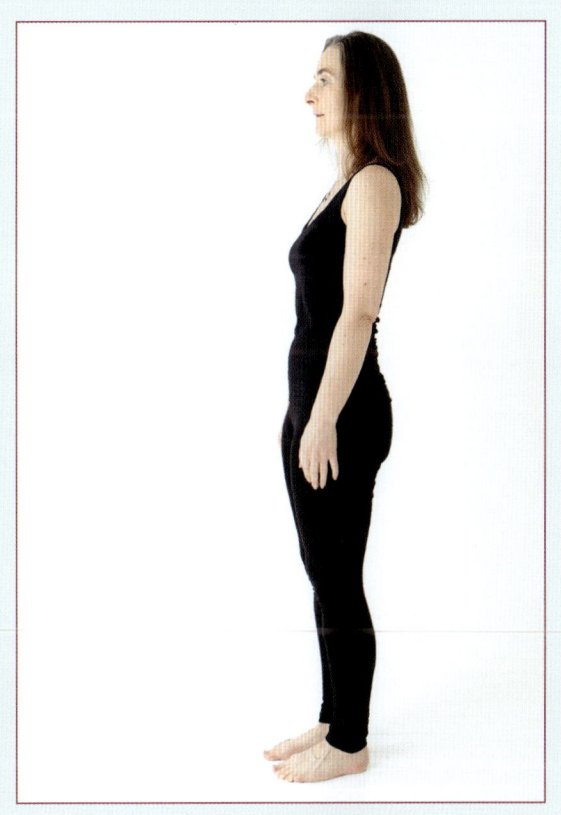

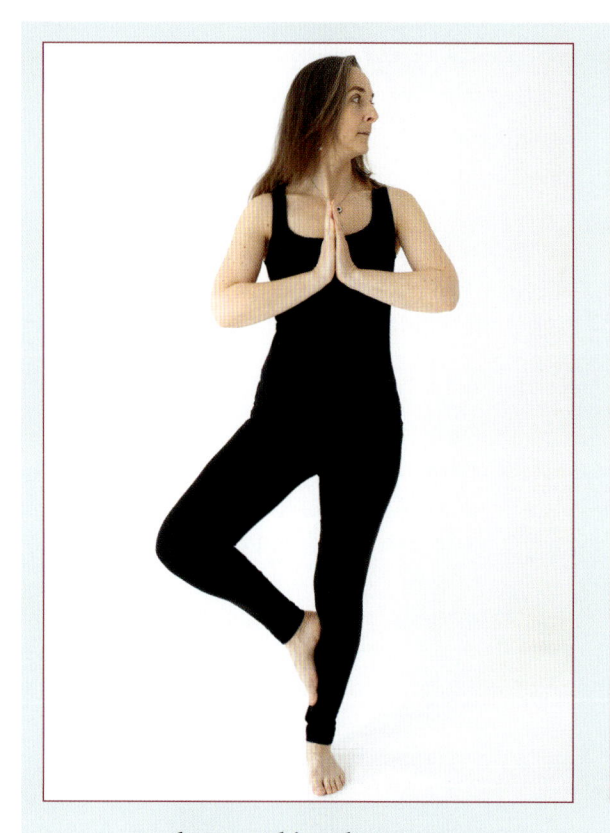

perhaps making the movement more sudden, or asking the student to look all around with the head moving (perhaps as if they are searching for a buzzing fly!).

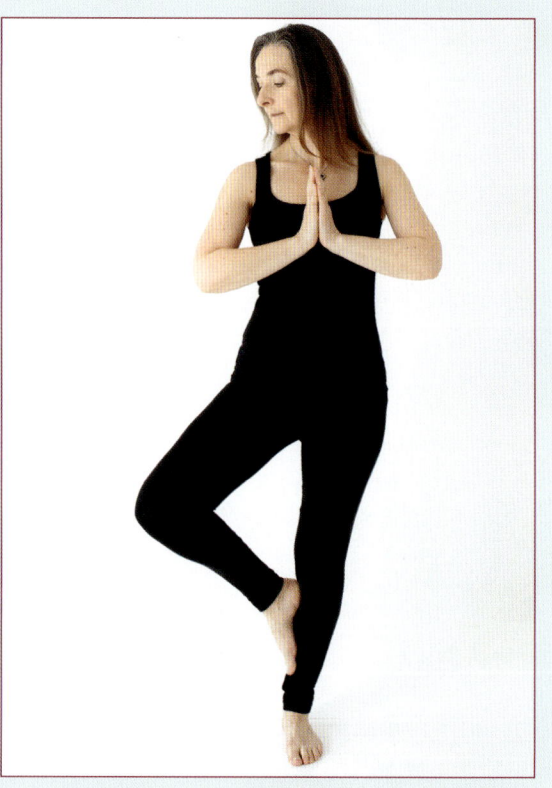

Always remember to use a wall for people with limited balance or osteopenia/osteoporosis.

Eye exercises

Our eyes are basically the only part of our brain that is visible from the outside. It is why specialists in neurology observe the eyes so closely. The brain is easily stimulated through eye movements. In particular:

- **Convergence:** Stimulates areas associated with posture, concentration, short-term memory (cerebellum).
- **Saccades:** Stimulate the frontal lobe and cerebellum, horizontal saccades awaken both sides of the brain and have been seen to improve memory (Parkin et al, 2023); vertical saccades stimulate areas of the brain involving posture.
- **Tracking:** Stimulates parietal lobe (which supports body mapping and proprioception).
- **Peripheral vision:** Stimulates PSNS (good for stress and anxiety).
- **Vestibular-ocular reflex (VOR):** This is when the head moves but the eyes stay fixed on one spot. Helps to reduce dizziness and vertigo, improving avoidance of falls.
- **Vestibular and visual together:** Aids balance.

1 & 2) Horizontal and vertical saccades in warrior. Saccades are quick rhythmic movements of the eyes up and down, side to side, or diagonally. They can be done without the hands to look at. Movements should be rhythmical and precise, as fast as possible, keeping up with your guided rhythm and changes of rhythm, until the eyes tire.

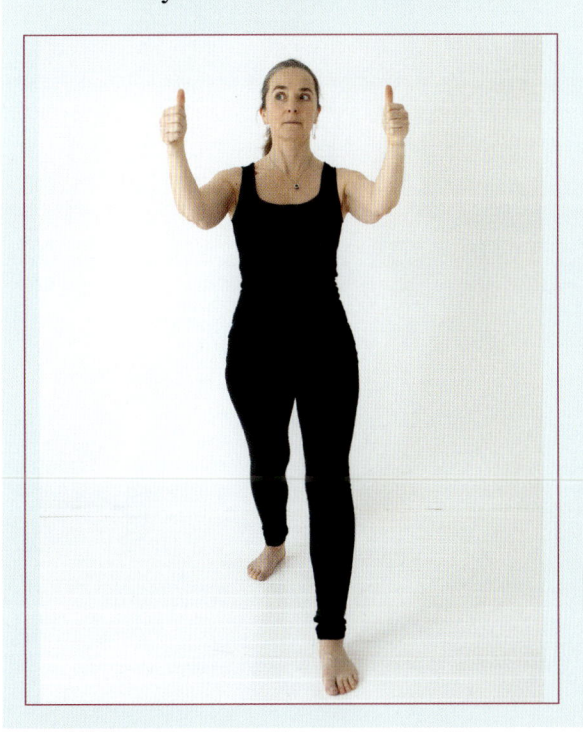

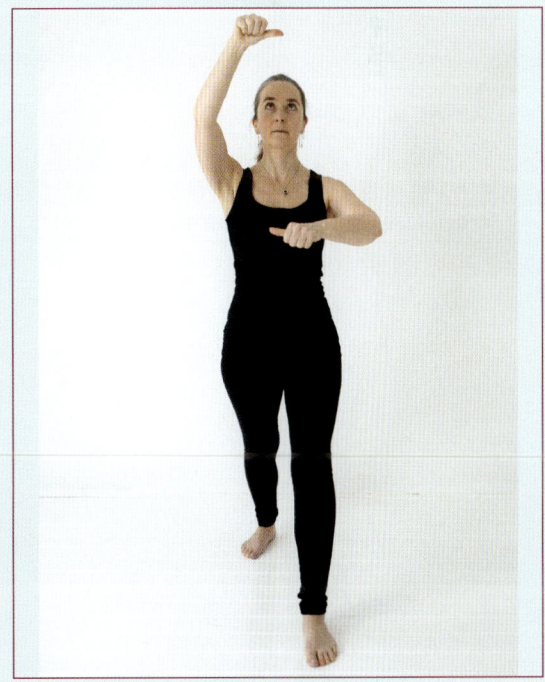

3) **Convergence.** Focusing on a small object, draw it toward the bridge of the nose and away again, three times. Focus with great conviction. Bringing it to the bridge of the nose is important, not the tip, as this stimulates the eyes differently than our usual habit.

A great bit of homework: Do it with your toothbrush after your morning or evening teeth routine.

4) **VOR.** Keep the eyes fixed on one point and move the head side to side or up and down. Develop speed while staying accurate. Could be done in warrior or in a balancing pose… carefully!

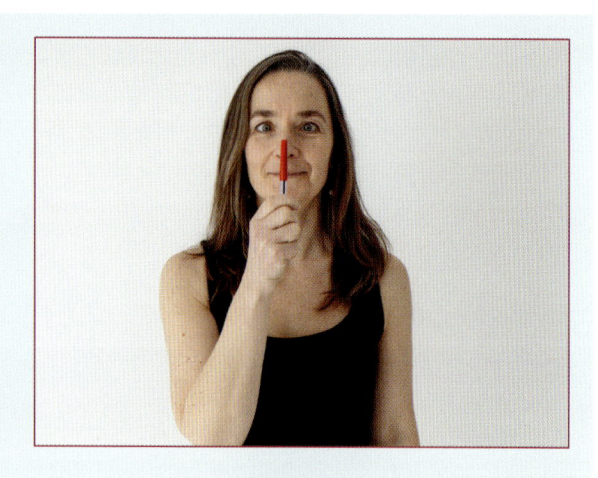

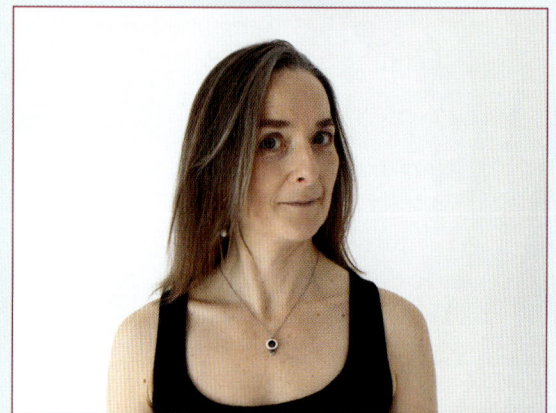

5) **Tracking** in trikonasana. Keep the head still and draw large circles with the arm, looking at the thumb with the eyes. Try to see the thumb consistently all the way around.

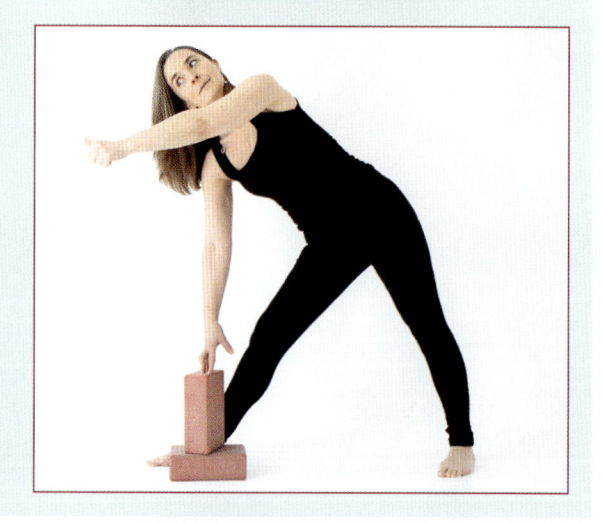

Nutrition

As with all body systems and organs, diet has a huge impact on the health of our brains. The "Mediterranean" diet is most widely suggested for the reduction of risks to brain health. In particular its abundance of fresh vegetables, olive oil, lean protein, and fish are considered valuable.

In addition, it is important to:

- Hydrate.
- Stabilize blood sugar which will mean fewer mood swings and energy slumps and to avoid insulin resistance which is a risk factor.
- Follow gut-health supports detailed in Chapter 5 b) on p.177, as the link of gut bacteria to mental health is well-researched.
- Consume foods rich in the "good fats" as low levels of Omega 3s have been linked to depression.
- Consume foods rich in B vitamins which support the feel-good hormones and energy production (richly available in molasses, nutritional yeast, meat, fish, dairy, eggs, nuts, beans, soy)
- Add berries and other deeply pigmented foods which are as important for our brain as they are for other systems.
- Remember that iron intake is important (eat oats, green leafy vegetables, lentils, beans, lean meat).
- Increase fruit and vegetables in the diet as studies show that those who consume more of them experience lower rates of depression. (Dharmayani et al, 2021)
- Enjoy nuts, seeds, and pulses which contain tryptophan, a building block of serotonin.
- Ensure good levels of anti-inflammatory foods (listed in Chapter 5).
- If it doesn't adversely affect you, have some coffee, even decaffeinated, which contains compounds that support neuro-transmitter health.
- Enjoy (assuming you do enjoy it) dark chocolate which has a high "hedonic" rating to make you feel good!
- Hydrate some more.

C) PELVIC FLOOR

The changing biology

The pelvic floor (PF) is not, as I used to visualize, one muscle like the breathing diaphragm, but a layering of muscles with fibers running front to back, side to side and diagonally (figure 4.3). It has a strong agonist/antagonist relationship with the breathing diaphragm: when we inhale, both diaphragms descend, and when we exhale they rise. Both support the breath, and the breath supports PF tone and relaxation.

Though men can suffer PF dysfunction, it is more common in women. PF health is a significant concern in women who have given birth vaginally, suffered physical trauma, and/or who are in postmenopause. Issues are widespread particularly, though by no means exclusively, among those older than 50. Pre-existing problems may begin to be more evident in perimenopause as there are many estrogen receptors in the pelvic floor and even the bladder, and the reduction of the reproductive hormones affects the PF in most women.

There is a variety of issues commonly referred to by the umbrella term genitourinary syndrome of menopause (GSM), covering everything from pain to urinary tract infections (UTIs) and thinning of the vaginal and vulval tissue (Angelou et al, 2020).

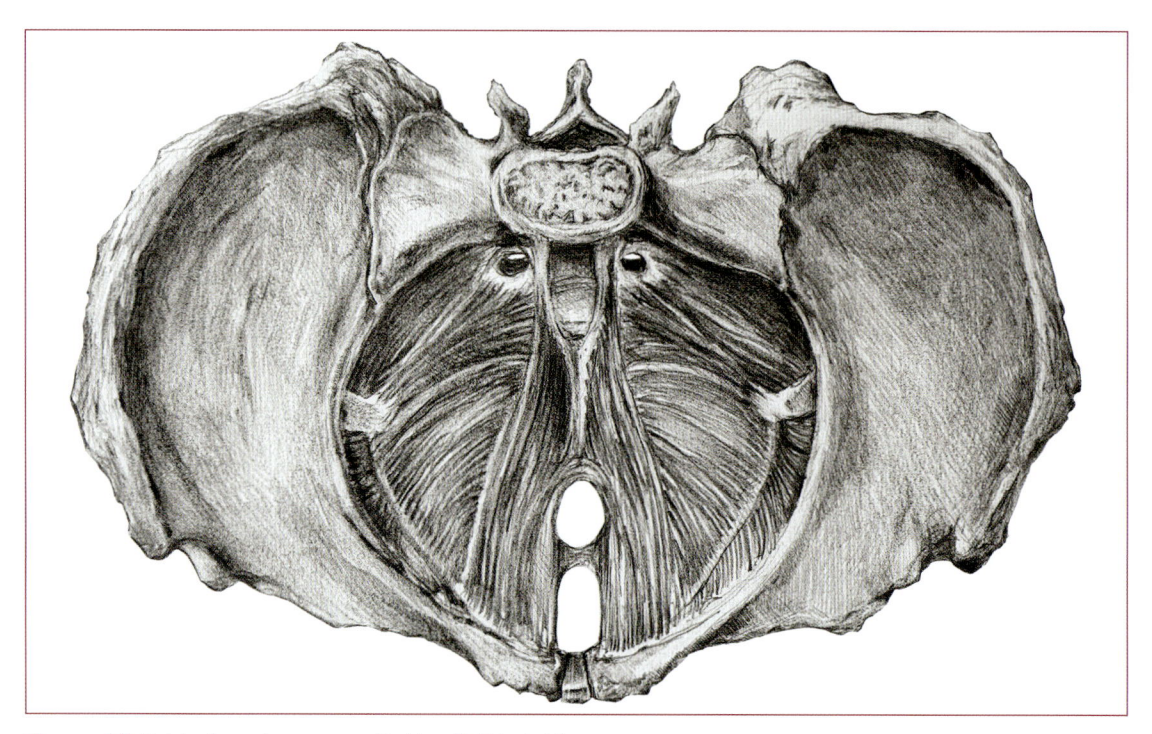

Figure 4.3 *Pelvic floor. Image credit: Henrik Frisch Kiær*

Why do so many genitourinary problems arise?

- Collagen deposition changes in the PF, vagina, and vulva, as in all tissues, decreasing strength, ability to stretch, and lubrication.
- The microbial environment of the premenopausal vagina differs from that in the peri/postmenopausal one. These microbial changes result in a higher vaginal pH, which increases the risk of the bacterial infections that cause UTIs.
- Dwindling estrogen can create an oversensitive bladder.
- Vaginal "atrophy" (thinning of the vaginal walls) increases the risk of UTIs.
- Reduced muscle mass and strength may exacerbate pelvic floor dysfunctions like prolapse and urinary incontinence.
- Low levels of strength are also common as we lose muscle mass, or indeed from the muscular fatigue associated with constant spasm.
- The likelihood of dehydration reduces the lubrication necessary for pain-free intercourse.
- PF spasm or tension can be present and cause pain and even urine leakage. Pain can exacerbate spasm, leading to more pain.

Now is the time to be proactive in strengthening and learning to relax the PF to reduce the risk of prolapse and/or urinary or double incontinence in later life, and indeed because reproductive tissue is less likely than other types to recalibrate after menopause.

Do we need to intervene? Some research is showing that if women are breathing well, with a free relationship between the respiratory and PF diaphragms, there will be sufficient natural tone and release to maintain health (Toprak et al, 2021). However, many women who have given birth vaginally will have had some sort of trauma to the PF which may or may not have resolved. Maintaining a healthy PF contributes hugely to quality of life. The changes in menopause can bring old issues to the fore, and menopause itself certainly has adverse effects, so though care from professionals specializing in PF may be needed, we as teachers should keep this area of the body to the forefront of our minds.

How yoga can help

When I ask my trainees the question "How can yoga help with the maintenance of the PF?", the first answer is often what you may be thinking: "Teach mula bandha" or "Teach strengthening exercises". But before we assume that strength is the only way, please remember that an overly strong PF is potentially as much a problem as one that is weak.

One of the possible causes of this is PF spasm. This can be due to clenching of the PF—as a result of painful intercourse, for example—which creates lactic acid. This can lead to a cycle of pain and further clenching, resulting in a state of chronic spasm, just like the more familiar vicious circle of, say, shoulder pain from tension creating more pain and so on. An overly tight PF can lead to an inability to begin to urinate, constipation, a sudden urge to urinate, and though it may seem counter-intuitive, can lead to incontinence.

So if your student has pelvic pain, bladder issues, UTIs etc., it's important that they go to a PF physiotherapist or a urogenital specialist for diagnosis before you recommend PF exercises. Likewise, it's worth sharing that there are symptoms that may feel like thrush or like UTIs that may not be due to these issues (which women commonly self-diagnosed and self-treated in their 20s and 30s), but to others that are more important to address. Any changes or symptoms should be checked by a doctor.

Now we can dive in!

Mula bandha

Mula bandha is essentially a PF lift, and its inward and upward focus is helpful for strengthening.

Many yoga teacher trainings don't instruct on or use this important tool, which is quite subtle, often refined to an isolated internal area (my own first teacher taught it as "drawing in and up at the cervix"). For our cohort, it should involve the urinary and anal sphincters as well as the vagina as we seek to protect against, or maybe even improve, prolapse of the bladder, intestine, uterus, and/or rectum.

Here are a few ways to help your student find mula bandha:

- Suggest a sense of drawing inward and upward at the cervix.
- If that is too subtle, suggest closing the walls of the vagina.
- If that's too difficult to feel, ask her to engage her anal sphincter in and up (or stop herself passing wind), then the same with the vaginal opening (or hold a tampon in), and then the urinary sphincter (or stop herself weeing).
- If none of that works, she could imagine picking a tissue up out of a box with her vagina.
- Lastly, just suggest for now that she stop herself urinating and passing wind.

Here is another way to help someone feel it:

- Have them sit upright on a chair, angling the pelvis so she can feel her pubic bones and sitting bones on the seat simultaneously.
- Possibly add in a rolled-up towel to straddle which may help her feel the area more clearly.
- Then suggest she try to lift the whole area of contact off the chair/towel.
- Ask her to try to continue breathing, as you will be asking her to use this lift during her physical practice.

The word 'lock' is often used to translate *bandha*, but this is unhelpful, in my opinion. It sounds too forceful and 100% effort is not helpful. The image I use is of the kind of effort we use when, say, holding a baby in our arms: we offer reliable support but without squeezing the precious bundle. This image of a gentle but reliable holding may increase her sense that her body needs and deserves detailed but gentle support.

Uddiyana bandha or hypopressives

There is some convincing research on the use of what is called hypopressive exercise/training to address PF prolapse, and core strength without risking intra-abdominal pressure that could exacerbate prolapse (Navarro-Brazález et al, 2020; Bernardes et al, 2012).

In my experience, a hypopressive "apnea"—as it is often termed—is just like uddiyana bandha, so uddiyana bandha could be a valuable tool for our cohort.

According to experts in hypopressive exercise, it is more effective for the front than the back of the PF.

The main difference between the apnea and uddiyana bandha is that the activation in the former is from a "false breath". That is, after a thorough exhale, you make the physical action of a lateral rib-expanding inhalation without actually taking in air. This creates the vacuum seen here.

In the traditional yogic bandha, the activation is sometimes instructed as a muscular drawing in and up of the abdomen (after a thorough exhale also). However I have seen uddiyana bandha taught as a false inhale also (but not, as far as I have read, in any older texts).

You can train as an instructor in hypopressive exercise (and a very similar technique called Low Pressure Training). There are now many physical shapes and movements taught while using the apnea, as in this half-wheel pose.

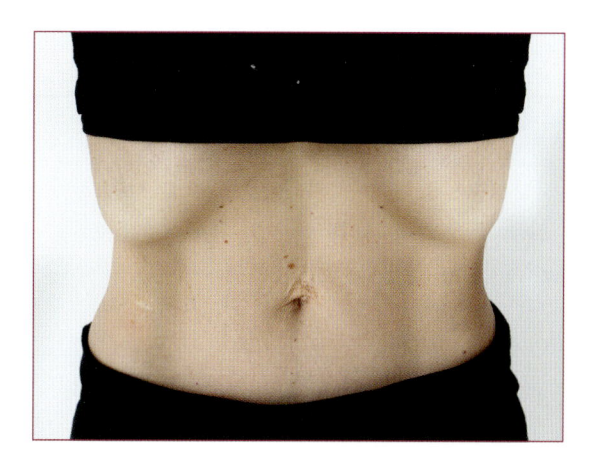

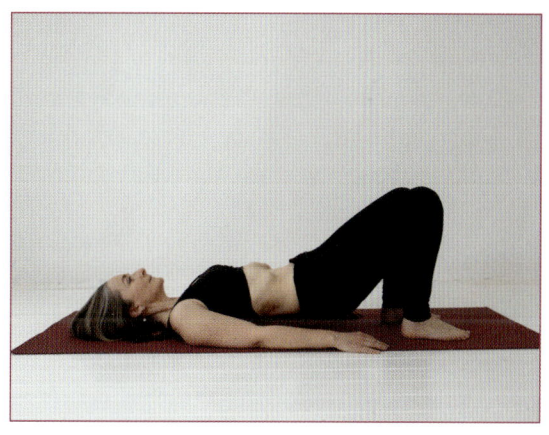

Teaching uddiyana bandha

This is best done a considerable time after eating.

When I was training, uddiyana bandha was taught standing, hinged forward at the hips, with hands braced on the thighs. Once we become adept at the lock, it can be done standing and in a number of postures, including that in the image above, or in downward-facing dog.

Exhale thoroughly.

> *In some yoga traditions the exhale is reasonably forceful, and may be pushed*

> *out through the mouth. If the exhale is not complete, it is very difficult to achieve the vacuum that is characteristic of this practice.*

Once all the air is out, consciously and dynamically draw the lower abdomen inward and upward. Imagine you are trying to tuck your navel up under your back ribs.

> *For beginners, a great adoption from the hypopressives way of teaching is that, after the exhale, you can hold your nose and take a "false breath," i.e. inhale without letting air in. This creates a lateral expansion of the ribs, which creates the vacuum that pulls the abdominal organs up toward the ribcage.*

> *This practice may create a closure of the glottis, resulting in a harsh inhale with a gasping at the beginning. If you relax your abdomen before inhaling, this somewhat stressful impact on the glottis can be avoided.*

Take some calm rest breaths before trying again.

This lock can be used during all postures, but that may be too much demand. Personally I teach a sort of baby uddiyana bandha by encouraging an inward and upward pull of the lower abdomen between pubic bone and navel. This won't create the vacuum, but give support via deep core activation.

I also consistently cue mula bandha during any postures that require strength.

Learning to engage the core

Look at the mighty transversus abdominis (TA) in figure 4.4. It is one of the main muscles of breathing, as it concentrically contracts on the exhale like a corset being tightened. It particularly engages when we exhale thoroughly.

At the same time, the pelvic floor contracts upward on the exhale, and relaxes downward on the inhale. As mentioned above, this is why full diaphragmatic breathing is such an important part of PF health.

There are many reasons why women in the stages of menopause would benefit from being able to connect to the TA and activate other core muscles. It can help:

- support effective breathing, which in turn supports the PF;
- stabilize the spine and help prevent falls;
- increase muscle tone, which can help with the metabolism;
- create better posture and good form if a woman is engaging in a weights program;
- help regulate the stress response.

Researchers are beginning to investigate links between strength in the core muscles and mental health and stress. There are neurons that control our adrenal response

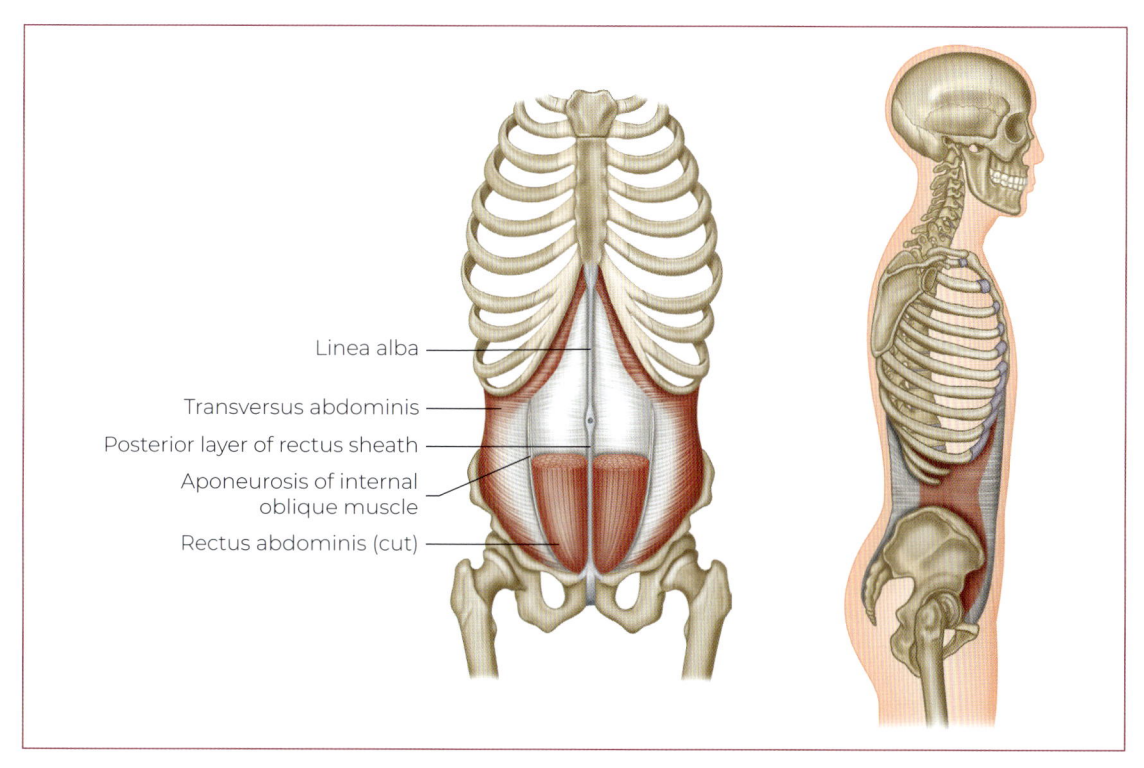

Figure 4.4 *Transversus abdominis (TA) wrapping around the torso*

in the same area of the sensory motor cortex that is responsible for our core muscles. Neuroscientists have hypothesized that this may be the link between exercise and better stress regulation. Overall, core strength is associated with reduced stress, anxiety, and depression (Cabanas-Sánchez et al, 2022).

So the practices in this core section could just as easily have gone in the section addressing mood changes (Chapter 5), or in the asana or bone health sections. I hope this will highlight the fact that, though this book has lots of sections, everything overlaps.

Exercises

Pelvic tuck

This is a supine version of cat/cow, but without the arching. Lying semi-supine, tuck the tailbone off the floor and press the lower back into the floor, without effort from the legs. Hold for 3–5 seconds (cuing avoidance of "bearing down"), then return to neutral. Build up the number of repetitions. Keep breathing!

Pelvic tuck with clock face

Imagine a clock face on your abdomen, with 12 at the top center, 6 at bottom center, just above the pubic bone. Arch and flatten the lower back a little, and press down toward 12 and 6 a few times, but with much less mobilizing, and more slow muscular control than a common pelvic tilt. Then imagine on either side of 6 on the clock, there are 5 and 7 o'clock.

Try to press straight down at 5 and then at 7 (or either side of the front of the pelvis), alternating side to side. It is a very subtle movement, with very little or no rocking of the pelvis or movement of the knees. This may help you feel and engage the diagonal fibers of the pelvis. Move slowly. Breathe.

Holding a block

Lie semi-supine with a yoga block at its second-widest between your thighs, and close to the knees. Exhale, tuck the tail, and grasp the block robustly.

Alternate between some repeated squeezing in rhythm with the breath, some faster pulsing, and some long holds.

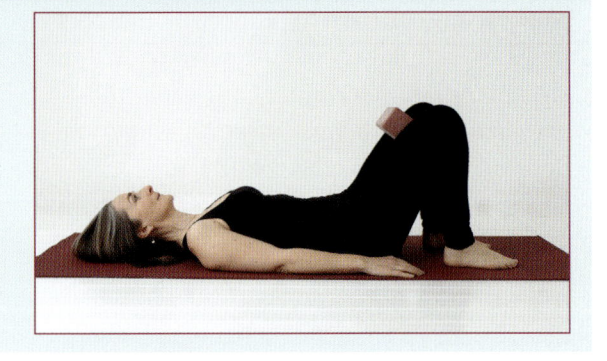

Raised leg block hold

This is a lot more tricky than the exercise above, and may be too much for people with lower back issues.

1) Lift your feet off the floor without rocking the pelvis.
2) Hold the thighs vertical, shins horizontal.
3) That may be enough, but you can add another layer of effort if you press your hands into your legs, and your legs into your hands.

As above with the block, but add engagement of mula bandha, and imagine a corset gently tightening around your waist (TA).

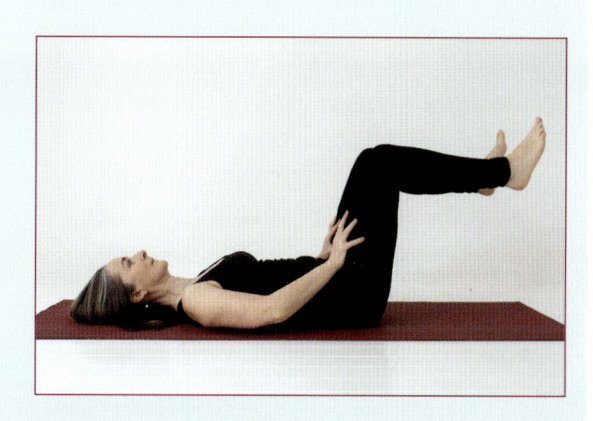

Cobbler

This is very effective to help you feel the PF and how the use of your feet affects it in different places.

1) Lie in cobbler pose, supporting the knees if it is immediately uncomfortable (but because this is an active exercise, it's not necessary for most).
2) On an exhale, press the soles of the feet together and notice that the legs and the PF engage. You may not notice how much is engaged until you feel how much relaxes when you inhale.
3) As you exhale again, press with just the heels.
4) Next exhale, press only with the balls of the feet.
5) Next exhale, press the outer edges of the feet together.
6) Next exhale, press the inner edges.

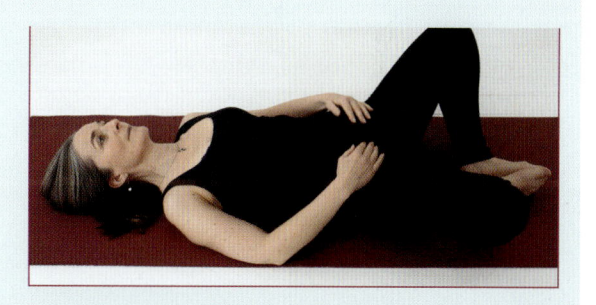

During each exhale, notice what area of the PF you can feel the most.

There is an almost infinite number of exercises you can offer. These are just some examples.

Relaxing the pelvic floor

In general, we all clench our diaphragms when we are in SNS mode, so any calming PSNS-supportive practices should help.

Breath practices

1) Simple diaphragmatic breathing, focusing on allowing the PF to move with the respiratory diaphragm.
2) A more targeted PF breath: Lie semi-supine, one hand on your belly. Inhale into the belly, allowing it to billow out. Move the breath down to the PF and, without pause, exhale and allow the air to move out without effort, as if the breath is moving out through the PF. Use as a meditation.
3) As you inhale, imagine your PF is a rose in bloom. As you exhale, imagine that rose closing gently to a Valentine's bud. Not harshly into a tight bud, but the perfect Valentine's bloom. As you inhale the petals bloom softly open. Repeat multiple times.

The bottom image is a version adjusted for people with possible issues/restrictions.

Do the above breathing practices in these poses:

Child's pose: Breathe into the back, relaxing the muscles around the tailbone.

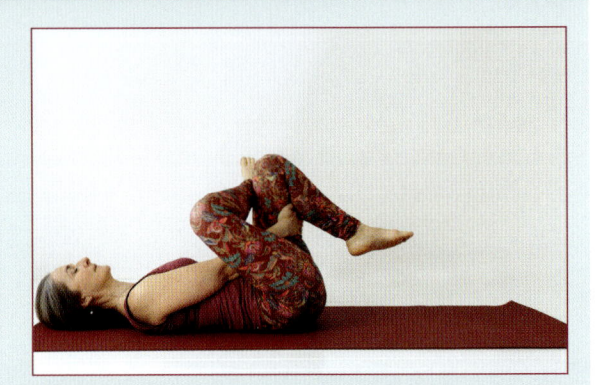

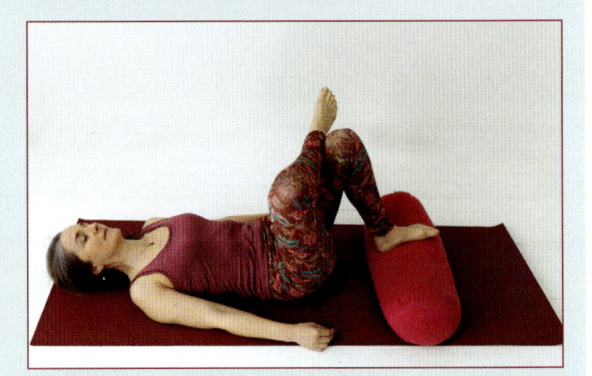

Reclining cobbler: see Chapter 3 e) on p.90.

Eye of the needle: A great pose in which to relax the PF.

Using core strength

Applying core connection and strength more broadly may give you opportunities to incorporate PF health and indeed a protective support to the spine. I encourage muscular awareness of the core in every posture where we are looking for strength or needing protection, especially for the lower back (and letting it all get nice and long and free in our restoratives!).

When effort is required, belly breathing is not advised. Instead, I suggest lateral breathing with continued 30% engagement of core musculature to ensure core stability, particularly when the spine is not supported by gravity (in warrior III, pyramid or side-angle pose, for example), or when the core is called on to move the legs. The psoas major (often spoken about in the singular, though there is of course one on each side of the spine), which lie either side of the lumbar spine and connect to the femurs, enabling us to articulate our legs toward and away from our body, are also an interesting point of focus in, for example, some of the supine work with bands.

Please be aware that with any engagement of the abdominal muscles we create intra-abdominal pressure. It's possible to unwittingly push down into the PF. Ensure you point this out to students and remind them to engage a gentle mula bandha or PF lift. Consider also suggesting to your students a mini uddiyana bandha. I often use the shorthand "mula bandha and uddiyana bandha" in the middle of the big list of other instructions!

The engagement of mula bandha and the core during practice should be at about 30-40% of our possible effort. The muscles involved have more slow-twitch than fast-twitch fibers, meaning they are built for stamina, not for intensity, and if we over-contract we recruit more of the more easily exhausted fast-twitch fibers. However, this applies when we are using these muscular engagements to support us over the course of a whole practice. In specific training of the PF we should include some fast engagement to train it to respond quickly when we need it (to avoid leakage when jumping, for example).

This stabilizing can't be sustained for a whole yoga class, which gives us more reason for little mini-breaks to relax the PF *during*, not just at the end of, the yoga class.

Staying connected

Apart from all the relaxing and toning and getting the PF checked, what about connection? Because of their fears regarding its changes, many women disconnect from their vulval and vaginal region. It becomes an alien landscape they don't want to visit.

In my teaching I try to ensure that the genitals are part of the picture when considering tissue that values movement and blood flow. So in a Yoga Nidra, for instance, I will include genitals or vulva in my body-scan. When describing what tissues are moving in cat/cow, I will mention these areas sometimes, as I might mention hips and spine.

Also, once I have the trust of a group, I would offer a practice like this, for mobility, for tuning in and making friends with your pelvic floor, hips, and genitals. Take time between each step.

- Organize a warm and comfortable place to lie down on the floor.
- Lie with your knees bent.
- Close your eyes if you're comfortable to do so.
- Become aware of your breath or the weight of your body for a few minutes.
- Then pour all your attention into your pelvis, hips, genitals, and pelvic floor.
- Notice that here are bones, ligaments, tendons, muscle, skin, and organs just like so many others areas throughout your body.
- Notice any sensations here; pulsing, coolness, warmth, tingling.
- Be aware of the millions of processes going on in the cells of this area of your body.
- Then notice if your hips and pelvis would like to move.
- Notice that movement can be tiny, imperceptible to the eye, but you can feel it.
- Begin to move your pelvis.
- You could rock it side-to-side.
- You could tilt it back and forth, arching and flattening your lower back.
- You could squirm it in circles.
- You could move it completely randomly.
- Now begin to imagine that you are a Hawaiian dancer in a grass skirt. Move your hips and pelvis as if you are trying to move that skirt to slow, sensual music.
- As you begin to allow free movement in your pelvis, let it increase and decrease again and again.
- Take your awareness to your hip joints. Imagine the movement is distributing unctuous oil throughout the joints.
- Take your awareness to your genitals. Imagine the movement is bringing blood flow to the tissues and moisture between them so they can slip and slide.
- Take your awareness to your pelvic floor. Imagine it opening into relaxation and closing into tone, like a flower moving from bloom to bud and back again.
- Let the movements reduce and reduce until they become imperceptible and eventually cease.
- Lie in stillness, resting your attention on the after-glow.
- Breathe.
- Rest.
- Take a good five minutes before you get on with your day.

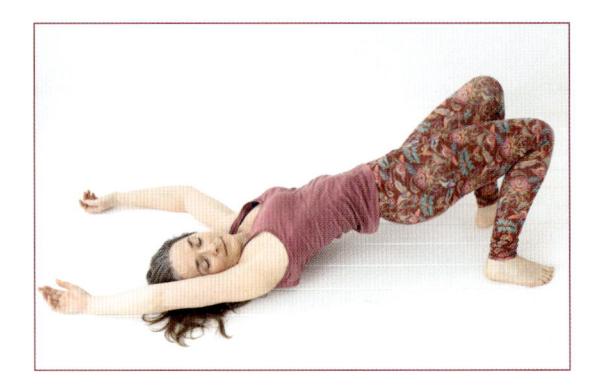

- You might want to mind yourself a bit extra today, knowing that you have allowed your body a freedom and expression that it may not have enjoyed in a while. If you're feeling vulnerable, perhaps spend some time in child's pose before you interact with anyone.
- Tune in to your nugget of strength.

Would you feel able to offer this?

Support outside yoga

Here are some important options to be aware of before we move on to our roles as teachers:

- Local estrogen in the form of pessaries, tiny pills inserted into the vagina, and/or cream is immensely effective and, as detailed in Chapter 6 where we look at medical approaches, so low risk as to be recommended even for women who can't take systemic MHT.
- Moisturizing: in particular, moisturizers with hyaluronic acid have been seen in one study to be almost as effective as localized estrogen (Chen et al, 2013).
- Lubricating (to avoid micro-tears during any sexual activity or exercising).
- Massaging to encourage blood flow.
- Self-pleasure to achieve orgasm, which supports PF health via blood flow (the frequency with which you would need to orgasm to build PF strength may be unachievable, so realistically, it's not the only route you need to take for strength).
- Vaginal dilators are also recommended medically for women with vaginal atrophy.

Avoid applying any creams with perfumes to your genitals. For lubrication, oils are a great alternative to perfumed creams and lotions found in pharmacies. These could include olive, avocado, or coconut oils. However, using oils too frequently may increase the risk of developing thrush.

Food for thought

Addressing PF health is a delicate area where language and trauma sensitivity (dealt with in the sections on emotion from p.163, and language, from p.46) are of great importance. But at the same time, sensitively using language that has hitherto been taboo may help to dispel the stigma and/or the lack of consideration given to genital health and connection. Is avoidance of words like vagina or vulva in a yoga class buying into shame or the sidelining of "women's issues" that has been the case in many spiritual traditions?

CHAPTER 5
A JOURNEY, SUPPORTED

In this section I offer you an array of additions to support women in the late reproductive stage, perimenopause, and into the decades postmenopause. While addressing symptoms and immediate and long-term health through yoga, you will also learn about ways to support a woman's journey in the latter half of her life through well-known lifestyle elements, including nutrition.

A) PERIMENOPAUSE, SYMPTOMS ADDRESSED

You can't alleviate menopause symptom by symptom because they are all interconnected, and for some symptoms and/or some women, only MHT will work. For others, unfortunately, nothing will work.

> When aiming to address symptoms, please be aware of three things.
>
> 1) You can't fix everything.
> 2) For the vast majority the symptoms of the MT are not so severe as to be a risk to life.
> 3) Other factors may also be at play: not everything a woman experiences in midlife—even if it's during the MT—is because of it!

Usually though, improvements are more easily available than many women expect.

Even simply by addressing areas of health, as detailed in the next four sections, we may see fewer or less severe symptoms.

For instance, it is possible to reduce symptom severity and frequency by supporting the pillars of health, which will maximize the possibility of reducing other contributing factors.

The four (or six) pillars of health are considered to be:

- Nutrition (and hydration)
- Movement
- Stress reduction and nervous system resilience
- Sleep.

You may also see connection and purpose listed as two further pillars.

Yoga for menopause prioritizes supporting these pillars of health to address health concerns and symptoms.

Sleep, hot flashes, and anxiety

I have bundled these three together because some of the researched complementary supports, namely paced breathing and CBT, have been seen to address all three. For all three symptoms, if a woman has been practicing paced breathing during the day when all is well, as outlined on p. 101, she can apply it as an intervention in wakeful moments, before bed, when anxiety is present, or at the onset of a hot flash. It may help her manage her experience and make it less distressing, as it calms the nervous system.

Ameliorating these symptoms in perimenopause is notoriously difficult. For example, though there is research showing that yoga can improve sleep, in the studies into perimenopause sleep improvements, the data are not as impressive for cohorts in perimenopause as for control groups in premenopause (Wang et al, 2020). What we *can* safely say, as with any intervention, is that yoga *may* help with sleep, anxiety, and the experience of hot flashes, and that we are adding tools which will further target this important area of wellbeing.

However, let's remember that science doesn't get everything right, and let me tell you that even my perimenopausal students have their best nights' sleep on the days they come to class. I have no doubt that *your* students report that they get better sleep on yoga nights.

Sleep

Sleep is one of the cornerstones of health. It is a detoxifier, a processor, a builder, and a healer. It reduces inflammation, it soothes the nervous system, it allows the brain to shrink so that it can be washed clean by the lymphatic system, and it is when a great deal of bone building occurs and muscle builds as the pituitary gland releases a growth hormone at night. Sleep is truly medicinal. Without it, we can do all the muscle and bone building and healthy eating and meditating we like, but lack of sleep will take a considerable toll.

Sleep disruption is one of the most common issues of perimenopause. I would bet my income that if women slept well in perimenopause, symptoms would be much less bothersome, and health risks would not elevate quite so much.

So, though short, this section may be this book's most important one.

Hot flashes and night sweats seem to be the first things that disrupt sleep for women and they continue to be the main culprits. When the body mistakenly thinks we are too hot, it wakes us, perhaps as a matter of survival instinct: *I must wake her so she can cool down!* This often results in a rush of adrenaline and cortisol and could be why many women experience anxiety or dread upon night-time waking that is associated with hot flashes or night sweats.

Even without hot flashes, we may see general and night-time cortisol levels that are higher than before perimenopause for many reasons (Fugate Woods et al, 2009). In part, this is because melatonin drops during perimenopause, so the possibility of getting sufficient sleep is significantly reduced. A lack of sleep will elevate cortisol levels (Späth-Schwalbe et al, 1992), and elevated cortisol disrupts sleep. The perfect storm.

Other possible causes of sleep disruption in the menopausal woman are:

- low progesterone
- blood sugar instability caused by impaired insulin function
- joint pain
- anxiety.

We can address many contributing factors, but we can't readjust the brain's new hypersensitivity to temperature which causes the vasomotor symptoms that are such central contributors. So while aiming to help your client with her sleep, not only is it disingenuous to make promises, but also if the suggested techniques don't reap dividends she may be hard on herself for not "doing it right" or come away with a sense of victimhood.

Practical sleep supports to suggest and/or teach

- Have a cool, or even cold, sleeping environment. In the absence of air conditioning, a silent fan may be necessary in warm weather. This may be the most helpful aid, given the temperature regulation issues. This can be tricky if a woman sleeps with a partner who likes a warm room, so it may be of value to consider separate rooms if their living circumstances allow. I have met many women whose partners are resistant to this because if feels like a relationship rift. But poor sleep has the potential to create relationship struggles and challenges our ability to see things clearly. It can heighten a woman's impatience, anger, and frustration, and may lead to a greater sense of relationship dissatisfaction than would otherwise be present. What I am saying is, separate rooms, far from being the death knell to a relationship, could save it.
- Limit evening light, including screens, as dwindling light stimulates melatonin production.
- Try to get exposure to daylight at intervals during the day: in the morning, to let the body notice it's morning, and in the evening light, so the body notices the sun is going down. This is related to the angle at which light hits the eye. Though looking toward the sun is beneficial for this intervention, never look directly at the sun.
- Let the light in the home be brighter, with more blue light in the morning, and lower (lamps rather than overhead lights) with more red and orange hues in the evening.
- Limit stimulants like caffeine and alcohol in the latter half of the day (these also often increase the frequency of hot flashes).
- Use CBT, detailed below.
- Nutrition and supplements can help, and some supplements have a good level of research around them, such as valerian, melatonin, and magnesium. However, it is important never to recommend specific supplements

- as some can interact negatively with some medications.
- Rest during the day to lower cortisol that may rise when we are running on empty. Far from hindering night-time sleep, a rest or nap before about 3 pm can support sleep for some.
- Legs up the wall is said to be a helpful pose for sleep. When we invert, our breathing naturally slows, signaling to the nervous system that we are safe. This is an achievable inversion for most (contraindicated in people with high blood pressure), whereas a headstand might not induce the feeling of safety, and a shoulder stand would be risky for many, especially those with lower than optimal bone density.
- Meditation or a restorative posture before bed have been seen to increase melatonin levels (Tooley et al, 2000) and serotonin. Both these hormones aid sleep. I would suggest that any relaxed pose, with deep breathing and a meditative state before bed should help to move us to the PSNS, which also supports sleep.

Hot flashes

Alongside night sweats, hot flashes—or flushes, as they are called in Ireland and the UK—are a significant part of the picture of this time. It's not certain what causes them, but it's thought that our body's temperature controls become more sensitized and a narrower range of temperature is tolerated. So our organism works to "fix" our temperature more conscientiously than it needs to. We become more temperature sensitive.

Hot flashes are not the same as night sweats, and many women experience them without any sweating. Night sweats usually manifest as waking up soaked in sweat with very little perceived change in temperature, and often becoming cold. Advice for night sweats is similar to that for hot flashes, but in addition, to have a change of pajamas right beside the bed and a few towels to sleep on so that, after a sweat, a woman can change without having to get up and turn on the light, and remove one towel and still have a dry one to fall asleep on, thus avoiding the need to get up and change the sheets.

Stress and anxiety can increase the frequency of hot flashes, perhaps because they tend to increase metabolic rate, which increases core temperature. There are widespread reports that alcohol, sugar, caffeine and even just eating can trigger a flash. Many women experience one immediately after waking. As well as a burst of adrenaline, there seems to be a relationship between hot flashes and cortisol. It appears to be a two-way street: the heat can trigger a stress hormone rise, and a stressful event can trigger a hot flash.

Perhaps surprisingly, it's not the sensation of heat that concerns some women the most, but the embarrassment that many report struggling with, particularly around appearance, and a sense of lack of control. Hot flashes, of course, also significantly disrupt sleep.

Practical supports

MHT can decrease the frequency and duration of hot flashes, some people find consuming phytoestrogen-rich foods helps decrease frequency (Chen et al, 2020), and it is accepted widely that CBT can be effective (Mann et al, 2012; Norton, 2015).

Yoga teachers cannot promise to stop hot flashes, but we can support the possibility of managing them with equilibrium.

It is worthwhile keeping a diary of what increases the frequency and intensity of hot flashes. There are more-or-less achievable ways to reduce most of the common triggers a woman may notice in her diary.

Personally, I find that a glass of cold water when I feel the subtle first signs that a hot flash is approaching can reduce the intensity, but only if I get to it quick. Once the hot flash has begun, it will simply take its own course. In me, those signs can be a tiny quiver of anxiety, like a gut feeling that something is awry, a little burst of nausea, or a moment of thirst.

They are frequent and tenacious companions which are sometimes, though rarely, with women for the rest of their lives. So, helping women change their relationship to these visitations can be transformative, and may be essential.

Begin with the possibility of "mindful hot flashes". Suggest that, if possible, when a woman feels a flash approaching, she pauses and watches the experiences in her body, tracking them and naming them. For example:

> *Here's the tingling in my cheeks. Now I can feel the heat in my arms. I am calmly removing my sweater. I feel the relief of the air on my arms. I'm noticing sweat coming on my upper lip. It's at its strongest now. I'm breathing with it. It's going to ease soon. It's easing now.*

I would even go so far as to say that one can develop a pleasurable relationship with these hot moments. Not all your students will be happy with this idea, and will need a big shift not to feel the dread and fear they harbor around hot flashes, so keep this under your hat, or make subtle prompts! But noticing what is happening can transform a miserable experience into something that is at least interesting:

> *What feels good about this all-over body awareness? What feels good about this water I'm drinking/taking off my sweater/ the air on my arms/the abatement of the heat/the coolness returning/the wanting to put my sweater back on?*

Sometimes I have loved a hot flash just because I know how yummy it will feel after it's done to pour the duvet back on my cooling body.

Anxiety

Anxiety is a very common symptom, and one of the first changes women in the LRS and perimenopause report.

Anxiety can arise spontaneously, with no perceived trigger, during and just before perimenopause. Unfortunately, these spikes can lead to anxious thinking, which in turn contributes to more chronic states. Anxious thinking tends to expect the worst possible outcome, and the individual often underestimates her ability to cope. Overworking, drinking, over-exercising, using diet to feel in control, or avoiding certain people are behaviors associated with an effort to escape the feeling of anxiety.

In perimenopause, anxiety may arise through a combination of circumstances and simple fluctuations of hormone levels. Understanding where it comes from, and seeing it objectively—*This sensation is the coursing of a hormone surge through me*, for example—can be comforting. You could suggest keeping a diary that details when the anxiety or anxiety-type sensations (like palpitations) occur. Some women will find a spike in anxiety, palpitations or nausea immediately preceding or after a hot flash, or upon waking. This may make it more evident that it is not caused by an alarming circumstance, and may be all a woman needs to let go of the worry associated with the feeling. In that diary she may also notice some external triggers like alcohol and caffeine, and also specific circumstances.

It may be helpful to remember that anxiety has its place in the tapestry of human emotion that makes us a successful species. Anxiety functions to keep us alert in new environments or situations until we know we are safe. Arguably, the entirety of perimenopause is such a moment—a long moment when there is such major change that our system keeps us vigilant. Our nervous system is keeping an eye out for any threats to be avoided or dealt with, until the system is used to, and less afraid of, the new environment.

Conversely, while recognizing the purpose of emotions or the requests they are making, sometimes we become too focused on an emotion, looking for logical reasons for its existence and making up reasons where none exist. Sometimes the emotions of perimenopause are simply biochemical: a burst of cortisol triggering anxiety, a hot flash triggering a release of adrenaline and a burst of dread, a drop in serotonin triggering low mood. Sometimes they are in keeping with a situation.

How to help

A question you could suggest she ask about all emotions is what their function is: *What does anger do for me? How does fear serve me? How does sadness support me? What does anxiety do for me?* This is the kind of inquiry that can be visited during restorative or Yin practices, perhaps using the TCM meridian element as a structure for your suggestions.

If anxiety is an emotion induced by a feeling of uncertainty or lack of safety in the nervous system (NS), instead of these behaviors you could suggest a woman inquire how else her NS might feel safe. A question to ask would be: *What are more self-caring alternatives that would help you feel safe?*

Perhaps:

- Permission to rest
- Sufficient nutritious food
- Seeking and acquiring appropriate help
- Reducing stressors
- Seeking community
- Putting in place whatever feels asked for by your symptoms.

You might be interested to offer her some of my favorite triage tools for when I have experienced anxiety:

Peripheral vision. When we are in SNS dominance our vision is quite blinkered. When we are in PSNS dominance, our peripheral vision is open. Practicing opening the peripheral vision can be very effective in inducing the PSNS. Simply look straight ahead and try to see as much as you can to left and right simultaneously. It can help to take your hands wide apart at head height and try to see them both while looking ahead. It's an easy one to fool ourselves with. Try wriggling the fingers to make sure you actually can see them!

Humming while orienting through my eyes (on p.163) and/or opening my peripheral vision has turned out to be the best collection of tools for me when I get a spike of anxiety.

If I use these techniques, my anxiety dissipates about 95% of the time. These two make up my personal cocktail of tools to support my nervous system. You can help your students find what works for them by introducing one or two suggestions of your own at a time, and teaching them repeatedly for a while, suggesting your student takes them home with her and practices them when she is not overwhelmed. Eventually you will have offered her a buffet to choose from, and she may find one or two things that are her lifeline.

CBT for sleep, hot flashes, and anxiety

In Chapter 2 I wrote about the use of cognitive behavioral therapy and how there is enough evidence of its efficacy to make it a tool recommended by mainstream medical and lifestyle professionals. Its benefits for sleep, hot flashes, and anxiety are particularly relevant for us. I recommend a document by Myra Hunter and Melanie Smith called 'Cognitive Behaviour Therapy for menopausal symptoms' (Hunter & Smith, 2017). You can share a link to it or print it out to distribute to your students. I have used this as a reference for years.

Sleep

CBT suggests that we try not to cancel activities the day after a bad night. Research shows this can increase worry about sleep, which can have a negative impact on sleep.

Try to change habitual thoughts:

- Turn *Tomorrow is a write-off* into *I will manage, I have before.*
- Instead of *I can kiss goodbye to sleep forever*, the thought could become *This is hard, but I know sleep can improve.*

There is a resource known as CBT for Insomnia (CBTI) that has some promising results for women in peri- and postmenopause. It can be accessed individually with a qualified practitioner.

Hot flashes

Consider changing these ways of thinking:

- Turn *Oh crap, here we go again, brace yourself for the horrors* into *Let's see can I do this one without panicking.*
- *I look awful* could become *I may be the only one who's noticing.*
- *When will this end?* could be replaced by *This symptom is going to gradually lessen.*

When worrying about others' opinion of you, ask yourself:

- *Is this thought or feeling true, kind, or appropriate?*
- *Do I judge others hot flashing in the same way I judge myself?*
- *Is seeing a hot flash as the enemy helpful to me?*

Whatever the negative thought, ask:

- *What is an alternative, kind thought, action or reaction?*

Anxiety

Because anxiety can lead to negative thoughts, which can lower mood and worsen the anxiety, CBT would suggest a woman asks herself:

- *Is this thought more negative than necessary?*
- *Is it overestimating how fearful I should be?*
- *Does it underestimate my ability to manage?*

Then consider:

- *Is this really a problem?*
- *If someone close to me was in this situation, how would I comfort them?*
- *Have I been through this and come out the other side before?*

Then check:

- *Is my reaction supportive to me?*
- *Did it make things better last time I reacted this way?*
- *If not, has there another approach that helped me?*

Further suggestions

Aside from CBT, consider identifying less personally with the sting of anxiety by, for instance, changing the language you use. Move from *I am anxious* to *I am having feelings of anxiety* to *I notice feelings of anxiety* to *I notice my awareness of anxious sensations*. Potentially this leaves us less personally affronted and more objective about the unwelcome intensity.

Another classic therapeutic tool is adding "and". *I am feeling anxious* **and** *I am walking*; *I feel vulnerable* **and** *I am capable*; *I am overwhelmed* **and** *later I will enjoy a book*. Notice these do not require momentous self-confidence, but they could involve self-appreciation: *I am nervous* **and** *I am a great colleague*; *I am feeling weak* **and** *I have friends who love me*.

These last few techniques are of course applicable to many emotional discomforts.

As anxiety, sleep disturbance, and sometimes hot flashes are often effects of an overwrought nervous system, any support for returning the NS to its ability to regulate itself (between SNS when required and PSNS when possible) is of value.

There is a very interesting clinical protocol called Organic Intelligence. According to organicintelligence.org, "Organic Intelligence® is a unique clinical practice of human empowerment, resiliency, and compassion, to resolve the impact of stress, trauma, and PTSD."

I am writing about this here not as a practitioner, but only from my own experience of being supported by an OI coach. As yoga teachers, we spend so much time looking after the wellbeing of others. I know we also need support. This is a resource I have found invaluable. It is one of the easiest ways I have found to let go of the stories that we sometimes tell ourselves that can add to our distress or discomfort. I highly recommend you look it up.

I share with you here some simple elements that I use, some of which are very much in keeping with aspects of yoga.

1. **Orientation practice:** In this technique, we align our attention to what feels good, or even just interesting. Maybe it's the breaking of light around the curtains or the softness of a blanket against the skin, or warm feet, or a cool breeze, a bird singing, or traffic in the distance. The idea is, through our senses, to allow our attention to notice something in our environment that feels good, pleasant, or okay.
2. **Eyes:** As she sits, suggest your student simply looks around and notice what her eyes rest upon and spends a little time looking at that thing. It could be a knot in the wood of a window frame, the angle where the wall meets the ceiling, the contrast between a pot plant and the window behind, etc. She can explore its angles, textures, light, shade, contrast. Do the same, looking around the room several times. This orientation can feel very comforting. Remember that vision is the sense the brain trusts the most. Our brain wants to feel safe. When we let it "see" where it is, it feels safe and we are able to relax into the PSNS.
3. **Connecting to the body:** After a moment of meditation, suggest she orientates, and then, if it feels okay, notice what feels good in her body (if nothing feels good, return to the orientation through the eyes, and indeed the other senses).

Please note that, via whatever practice that we may offer, developing deep levels of interoception can be very challenging. As a teacher, I often suggest number 1 as a practice during a sleepless night or upon waking and feeling low or jittery. I often use number 2 as a way of bringing students back to the room after a meditation or Yoga Nidra.

I found the orientation practice transformative during the worst sleep disruption of my own perimenopause.

This is my interpretation of this work which was developed by Steve Hoskinson. You can find out more on organicintelligence.org.

Changing mood

As well as anxiety, most women, at some point in their perimenopause, experience one or more of the following:

- Low mood
- Increased anger
- Lack of joy
- Libido changes.

There are many estrogen and progesterone receptors in areas of the brain that affect mood. The unfamiliarity of the sensations of perimenopause can make us fear the worst, and create a knock-on effect that does not serve our mood. All of these states can be exacerbated by poor sleep; lack of joy and loss of libido can be exacerbated by low self-esteem, and low mood by feelings of embarrassment and feelings of loss.

The tendency can be to withdraw from connection because a woman may be afraid of showing up with "unsavory" behavior. Withdrawing will take her away from company at a time when company can boost the feel-good hormones, give her a sense of shared experience, make her feel she's not alone, and provide her with tips for handling her situation. CBT advocates trying to look at things from a broader perspective by noticing the things in your life that you value. Low mood or low self-esteem can contribute to our tendency to drop out of things we love. An open, bright, "all is welcome" yoga class, rather than one with a rarefied atmosphere of reverent calm, could make your student feel she is more acceptable to you and, slowly, to herself.

In a bright and playful class, can we allow a woman's emotional life to be represented even on the mat? Can we allow emotion *into* her practice so that yoga is not about "letting your worries float away" at a time when that feels much less possible than hitherto? Can we practice, or offer practices, in ways that validate her feelings?

I think we can, and we should. Here's how we might go about it.

Honoring mood

You could lead your students in this simple standing warm-up:

- Swing the body as if trying to see behind you on both sides;
- Swing the arms, with a nice rhythmic, dynamic motion that twists the body and brings the arms into contact with the back;
- Swing the arms upward to the sides (like a golfer);
- Trot up and down the mat on different edges of the feet;
- Offer a physicalized breath with a vocalized exhale (the breath of joy).

Avoid swinging upside down for people with osteoporosis, lower back issues, glaucoma, or high blood pressure.

This warm-up lends itself to the following mood-honoring additions:

- As you lead them, offer a suggestion for each woman to move as if she is a kid who wants everyone to know how she is feeling. (In cueing the feelings, leave out anything too triggering, like anxiety or rage, that we might not be able to support in a busy class or online.)
- Encourage them to make sounds. This can be difficult but it is worth helping women find the bravery to express themselves and be heard.
- Keep it light with some playful offers like: *Do this movement as you are feeling now, then imagine you are:*
  - *really tired*
  - *full of energy*
  - *feeling strong*
  - *frustrated/grumpy*
  - *bored.*
- Ask them to notice what it's like to give themselves the option of expressing the emotion rather than wishing it away. Does it stay? Amplify? Move on? Does it feel like a reasonable reaction or is it out

A JOURNEY, SUPPORTED

of balance with the stimulus (the "why" of the feeling)? You and they may notice that when we give the feeling space to express itself, it shifts or burns itself out.

- Be sure to take control and move on at some point:
  - *Okay, see if you can let go of that practice and bring your body to stillness. Take a few lion breaths, and imagine you are spitting out that feeling. Then bounce it out, draining it into the earth. Now wiggle and shake. Wobble your flesh. Feel the fun of that ...*

Shifting mood

Sometimes it's not possible to be with our mood, to sit with it, honor it, or even tolerate it. Anything that engages the mind fully can help us move away from getting involved in the story of the emotion or energy we are feeling. So, we can give the brain something else to do, like some of the brain-training exercises. Try this one:

1) Hold your hands out in front of you, palms down.
2) With the dominant hand (the one you naturally write with) flap the palm up and down rhythmically.
3) This is all that hand will do, and it should not stop or lose the rhythm.
4) The non-dominant hand now begins to circle from the wrist (not the whole arm).
5) Then reverse the circles.
6) Don't allow either hand to imitate the other.
7) Once you manage the flapping and circling, try drawing figures of eight with the non-dominant hand.
8) When you master that, reverse the eight or try a sideways eight (infinity symbol).
9) Then draw your name in the air with the non-dominant hand.
10) Then the alphabet. And backward!
11) Then do the whole thing with feet instead
12) Then feet and hands together!

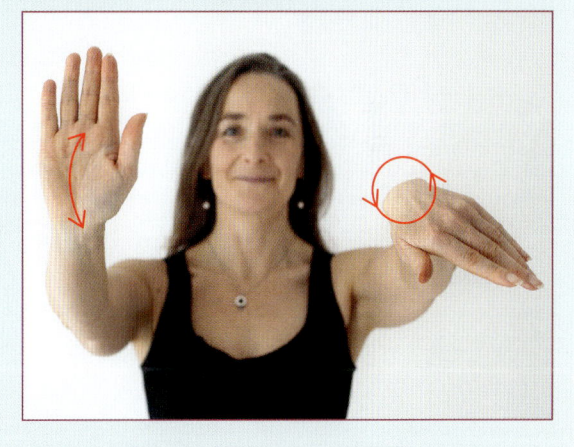

(Only add these last three after the others have been mastered.)

Soon the emotion will be a thing of the past!

This is a great way to show your students that there are many ways to meditate, if one-pointed attention is the aim of meditation. I teach this exercise in the teacher training, and suggest its use for brain-food as well as mood. You can do it with hands during a seated practice, or hands and feet while sitting in a functional staff pose. It has great ongoing value as you can start with the most basic movement and add challenge after challenge over weeks, as listed.

We can show how to use postures or practices to build our coping strategies when it's not optimal to let our feelings dominate a moment—when we are caring for someone or in the middle of a job interview, for example!

- Instead of performing that warm-up expressing her grumpiness, etc., offer her the possibility of moving as she would *like* to feel (or as she feels she needs to feel to get through the challenge for which she needs resilience). This works nicely with sun salutations: *Do this round as if you have all the calm, strength, and/or enthusiasm you need.*
- Teach some postures that embody, to you, some of the feelings you expect may be desirable, like strength (warrior I for example), calm or pleasure (maybe a somatic movement), enthusiasm (dancer maybe), patience (sitting still), self-expression (that playful standing warm-up). Ask the student to see if these postures do engender these feelings, or if not, what positive feelings do they conjure for her.
- Ask her to think of a posture that makes her feel good, and to perform it (maybe one you have just taught, or another of her choosing). Suggest that she performs it consciously, and exaggerates what feels empowering or good about it. She could see if this changes the way she inhabits the posture, if it changes her facial expression or thoughts. Suggest that it may be possible for her to imagine herself in that posture when in the middle of a situation where she needs that quality. Above is an image of me doing my "Don't mess with me, I'm holding up the world" version of warrior I!

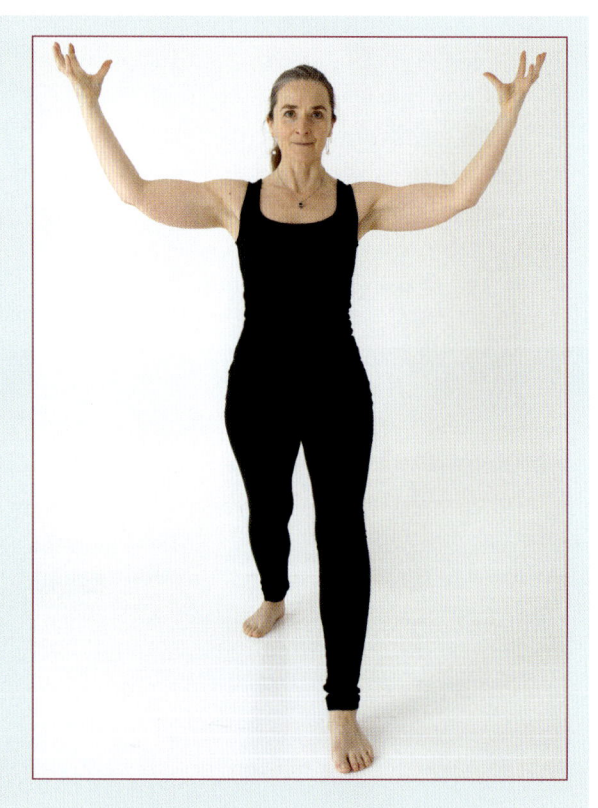

Outside-in

It is possible to temporarily shift our emotions from the outside in when we don't have time to do postures, or to engage in a session of positive self-talk.

The following is an exercise inspired by research into "voluntary facial action" where we bring onto the face the expression of that which one would prefer to feel, rather than what one is feeling. This has convincing results for immediate relief or reduction in intensity of mood (Söderkvist et al, 2017). I take it a step further, adding cues for awareness of how the whole body reacts to the shift in facial expression.

Give each of these suggestions time to materialize.

1) *Stand or sit neutrally.*
   - *Think about a moment when you were glum.*
   - *What would the expression on your face be?*
   - *What shape would your mouth take?*
   - *Your forehead? Your eyes?* 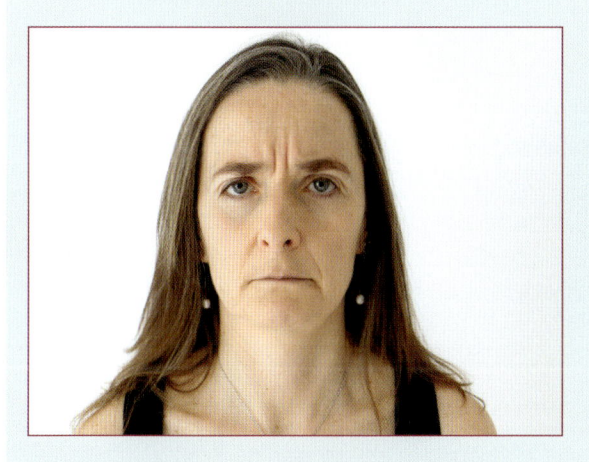
   - *How does that affect your shoulders and spine, your whole body?*
   - *How is your mood now?*
2) *Think about a time you were delighted.*
   - *What does your mouth do? Your eyes?*
   - *And your spine? Your hands?*
   - *Exaggerate how your physical body changes.*
   - *How is your mood now?* 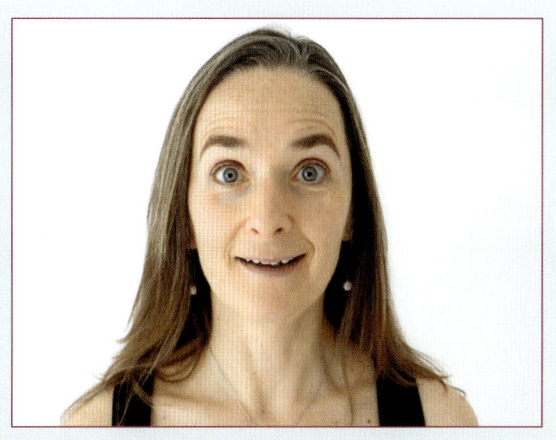
3) *Now remember or imagine a moment you felt really calm, at peace. Envisage the moment.*
   - *What is the shape of your mouth?*
   - *How do you feel around your eyes?*
   - *What position are your hands in?*
   - *How does your spine sit?*
   - *How is your mood now?*

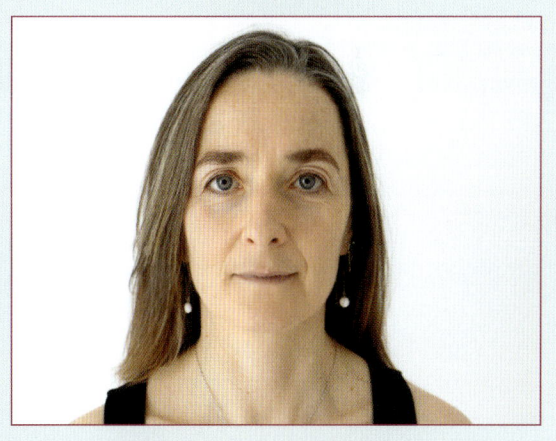

Again you see how I have not gone into major emotions. You may choose to play with others—tired, energized, happy, etc.—but I tend to keep it playful, so as not to trigger, but also so as not to undermine emotions that deserve space to be known and attended to.

Note that this is seen to work in the moment of intervention rather than as a long-term support. It is a handy tool when a person just needs a quick fix when the way she is feeling can't be given time and may need to be set aside for a moment.

Energy and focus

The next three symptoms often feed into each other, and much of what which supports one will support the others.

Fatigue

You can be reasonably sure that most of your students have too much on their plate, and many may be over-exercising, possibly undereating, and sleeping badly. But although it is often due to the more obvious causes, fatigue may be tricky to address because it can be related to many other things. It can be caused by hypothyroidism, stress, low iron, reduced lung function and many other issues that can be part of, or independent of, perimenopause. Getting blood tests to rule out reasons other than perimenopause and/or life-load is advisable.

What you can offer

Firstly, in your circle sharing time, when responding to students who bring this up, you can talk about the effects of perimenopause that can lead to fatigue. Gentle nudges to get an all-over health check-up and blood tests would not go amiss, and perhaps advising a visit to a nutritional therapist. In my work in nutrition, I notice that many women benefit from small dietary tweaks that can make a considerable difference to energy.

Remind your students that:

- The way their bodies handle exercise may change (Chapter 3 d) on p.70–71).
- Endurance exercise is not as menopause-friendly as shorter cardio sessions and strength work.
- Rest after exertion is always important, but now more than ever.
- Perimenopause is a nutritionally demanding time.
- Without sleep their body needs more rest.

Overwhelm

Overwhelm is a word you will see in lists of perimenopause symptoms. When I went to get a check-up and blood tests to determine why I was feeling as I was during what I suspected was early perimenopause (I was right!), my doctor asked me if I was experiencing acopia. I had never heard the word before, but it was so apt in describing what I was feeling, I cried with relief. Many feel this term pejorative, but I found liberating!

Acopia is a term used in some medical situations to describe the condition when someone is compromised—by illness, for example—and can't manage normal life, particularly socially and mentally. Perimenopause is not an illness, but it can leave us feeling vulnerable or compromised in the way that illness can.

Overwhelm is often a companion to fatigue. It is another symptom the cause of which can be hard to pin down. Yes, estrogen acts as a buffer for the brain against stress, and progesterone is a calming hormone. But also, life is more constantly demanding than most nervous systems are made to handle.

I feel the main way to deal with overwhelm is to have less demand placed on us. The only way we can do that is by recognizing our capacity and then advocating for ourselves by saying *no* more often than we have in the past.

I have lately been considering the possibility that we are not, in fact, *less* capable during and after perimenopause, but that before, in our adult years, we were incapable of recognizing our *true* capacity. The average age of burnout in the workplace is 32. That's nothing to do with perimenopause, and everything to do with taking on too much for our system to handle.

I often wonder what perimenopause would be like if we:

- were valued for something other than our productivity
- didn't think we had to be fabulous, but just enough
- hadn't already pushed ourselves to depletion
- lived in an inter-dependent community
- had already learned to say no
- didn't mind if people thought we were unwilling or selfish
- recognized our equality with others, and that someone else can do what we have thought only we could.

What you can offer

Perhaps sharing the perspectives above during a talk or as content of a meditation might be empowering. Overwhelm is essentially nervous system dysregulation from too much input, so any strategies that support the vagus nerve could be taught in ways that make them accessible and achievable.

The expectations meditation in Chapter 3 is aimed at this struggle.

Brain fog

Brain fog is very much connected with fatigue and overwhelm, and much of what is needed to handle overwhelm will help us to cope with brain fog too. Hydration is immensely important for the brain, as is regular fuel from food throughout the day. A simple quick trick to help concentration is to drink cold water.

Brain fog is one of the most common issues reported during the stages of menopause, and is especially concerning if women begin to feel they can't rely upon themselves in their work. Most of the people I have worked with who have found a way to manage life with brain fog have done it by putting strategies in place like ensuring someone at work knows they may need extra reminders, or by delegating things that they know can be done by someone else.

The most distressing parts of brain fog for me were forgetting to turn up to teach the same class three times in one year, and forgetting to do things like turn off lights or set the alarm in a studio I was renting, multiple times.

The only way that I was able to improve these things was by giving myself space. I would stop before rushing out the studio door on to the next thing, and double-check. I put multiple reminders in my phone as to where I needed to be. I apologized to the people involved and told them what was happening. In one instance that led to my being asked to give a talk about menopause to the entire company, a great result! But in another instance I ended up choosing to leave a studio I was renting because I felt misunderstood and embarrassed, as my mistakes looked like, and seemed to be interpreted as, carelessness.

Why do I tell you this? To illustrate that, though we can help, a) we can't fix everything, and b) not every outcome is bad—or good.

What you can offer

- I have had some success with the brain-training techniques detailed in Chapter 4 b) on p.132–140. Practicing convergence and saccades with the eyes have helped some clients with focus in the middle of the day.
- Keep your students alert by not allowing them zone out in class: create memory challenges like teaching a short flow of postures on one side, and then ask them to perform it on the other side without your instruction.
- Meditation is known to improve memory and concentration.
- Focus to a great degree on assisting sleep improvements.
- Again, the value of rest is considerable, as is any nervous system support.

Further supports

You can further help ameliorate fatigue, overwhelm and brain-fog by:

- Teaching gentle, somatic-style classes where *pleasure*, rather than strength or effort, is the main aim
- Using language that implies the value of *softening* rather than pushing through
- Teaching simple deep breathing skills to help with lung function and oxygenation
- Offering movement snacks (swinging arms, running up and down the stairs, any stretching) or brain-stimulating snacks (detailed in the section on brain health) that can boost energy at a time when women need to just get through the next moments/hours
- Supporting their resting skills by offering women meditation or breathing or restorative yoga techniques (aka "rest snacks").

Rest snacks could be:

- Restorative poses—many can be done without a warm-up, and it's fine to snooze during a pose!
- A nap in the afternoon—it can be a true lifesaver, and for most it doesn't interfere with sleep if it's not too long or too late
- Yoga Nidra in the afternoon
- Drinking tea mindfully: Stop everything, make tea and sit with it away from work or even away from a book, and notice the feel of the cup, the temperature, the smell and color of the tea, the sensation of the first mouthful. Stay with this simplicity for the entire cup
- Staring at the sky
- Standing in the middle of the floor and counting backward from 90, or even just 25!
- Ujjayi breathing in the car for five minutes before going in to work/a busy household

- Alternate nostril breathing at your desk: I tend to teach this without the retention, or with a very short one. It can even be done without closing the nostrils, simply with the thought of isolating the breath in one nostril.

Aching joints

Women often find that their healthcare professional can't figure out what's wrong in the case of aches and pains, and some have been misdiagnosed with fibromyalgia during perimenopause. Where joint pain is body-wide or on both sides (bilateral) and/or there have been investigations to rule out structural issues, aching joints are sometimes a result of somewhat higher systemic inflammation than before.

Inflammation is the body's response to, among other things, any sort of stressor like an injury, to chronic stress, alcohol, smoking, auto-immune disease, foods that the system can't digest, and over- or under-exercising. You may notice that inflammation is not listed as a symptom of perimenopause, yet research points to elevated levels for markers that denote inflammation in the blood compared to premenopause (Malutan et al, 2014). Estrogen is anti-inflammatory, and impacts the feel-good hormones, some of which are also anti-inflammatory, so their lack may also be a contributing factor.

This illustrates that symptoms may not be caused directly by the fluctuations in the reproductive hormones, but by more systemic effects of the pressure this change places on the body. So, the *symptom* of achy joints may be caused by *inflammation*. This may seem like semantics, but it has a practical application: there are interventions that individuals can investigate in order to reduce inflammation, even if they are not raising estrogen and progesterone levels through MHT.

What you can offer

On a local level, as teachers caring responsibly for joints and fascia, we should reduce the risks of encouraging inflammation through repeated excess stress or injury by avoiding externally forced stretching at full range of motion, and avoiding the idea that postures have a sought-after end point.

Add variety to your classes. Repeating the same movements over and over is less than optimal because it leads us away from variety of movement, which we know is much more valuable for heart, brain, muscle, and bone than repetitive action. It also leads to more wear and tear and RSIs (repetitive strain injuries).

Suggest movement in bed before getting up. It can help to warm synovial fluid, get neurotransmitters up and running, and enliven stagnant tissue so the body is ready to perform the tasks of getting out of bed. This can reduce that stiffness of gait in the morning as we clamber out of bed. Some women report "feeling old" in the morning. This can lead to low mood or depression, which can then contribute to inflammation in a self-perpetuating cycle. So this morning movement snack encourages a positive cycle.

As well as potentially injuring joints, the way a woman exercises can deplete her energy and create inflammation which may not resolve as readily in perimenopause. You may be interested to watch the video 'Rethinking Exercise when Perimenopause Makes it Difficult' in my YouTube free resources.[3]

Happily, when we address joint pain through reduction of inflammation, we may also be addressing much broader issues, as you will see later in the section on protecting health.

Weight gain

In the course of our lifespan, the shape of the human body changes from that of a baby to that of an elderly person. These changes are normal, and we expect change from baby to toddler to child to prepubescent to teen to adult, even from midlife to old age, and would be worried or confused if change did not occur. But this does not seem to apply to the natural changes in body shape for women in midlife, as they move from the menstrual years to menopause.

You will see a lot of conflicting opinions about why women's weight tends to increase in perimenopause. Some say it's related to slowing metabolism as a result of loss of muscle mass, some that it's because women feel more fatigued so they move less, some that estrogen regulates the processing of lipids (fats) and glucose (higher blood sugar causes the liver to convert and store glucose as fat).

What we definitely see is that the ways in which women have controlled their weight seem no longer to work. However, it is true that, for most, the simple logic still applies: the only way to reduce weight is through a calorie deficit (fewer calories consumed in relation to energy expended).

But this is a time when a woman's body needs rich nutritional input because of the decreased support of estrogen and progesterone, particularly related to muscle, bone, brain, and heart health. In addition, after menopause estrogen is produced by your adrenal glands and by your adipose tissue (fat), so some degree of increased adipose tissue may support estrogen levels postmenopause.

But because of societal preferences, the majority of women feel pressure to fight the natural changes in body shape. Therefore, they often choose to drastically reduce their food intake in an effort to stave off these changes at a time when adequate nutrition may be more important than ever.

Bear in mind that:

- As well as not meeting her increased mineral, protein, fat, and complex-carbohydrate needs, dieting (at any age) can induce the stress response, creating blood sugar imbalances. When blood sugar crashes, cortisol is released.
- Cortisol leads to increased appetite, in particular quick-fix cravings often for refined carbohydrates. We can see why, by upping exercise and reducing food intake, a woman may unwittingly be increasing stress in a way that creates the conditions for further weight gain.

---

[3] Available at www.youtube.com/watch?v=Khyk6OCigCw.

- Cortisol is "catabolic". Essentially it consumes bone and muscle tissue, leading to all the associated risks of osteoporosis and to a slowing of metabolism which may lead to weight gain.
- The calorie restriction protocols of many weight-loss diets usually end in the laying down of fat to a greater degree once calories are reintroduced.
- The considerable potential negative effects of drastic diets that restrict calorie intake or that restrict food groups are discussed in Chapter 6.

Regarding concerns about health in relation to weight, in my nutrition coaching I tend to address how my clients are *feeling* in terms of energy, sleep, digestion, and mood. Often when these are addressed the person feels so much better that they lose their obsession about their shape as they are too busy enjoying how they feel. I aim to aid women to enjoy health at a broad range of sizes, without assuming the need for all to conform to a specific body-mass index. This is because we know that many positive signs can be seen in the blood tests of people who improve their habits of movement, nutrition, and stress regulation, even if this does not result in weight loss (Bacon & Aphramor, 2011).

Blaming weight for health issues is a simplistic view of a complex situation, and we know that healthy weight is on a spectrum. It is possible to be lean and unhealthy, large and healthy, and dangers exist at both ends of the body size spectrum. A fascinating paper by a group of professors of medicine talks about the risks to health of "fat phobia" and how the medical world could do with rethinking its approach (Sturgiss et al, 2017)

What you can offer

De-stigmatizing what women may consider excess weight can be done by pointing out the benefits of adipose tissue: it is sensual, replete with lymph, creates a small amount of estrogen, and we can be healthy in bodies of all sorts of shapes. However, if a woman is struggling with unwelcome weight gain, we can support her desires to become more comfortable in her body. What worked for your student before may not work now. So, what might help her?

- Teaching her stress regulation techniques
- Supporting her muscular strength to improve metabolism
- Helping support her sleep
- Helping her develop interoception so that she can be:
    - aware of her energy and how much exercise is enough
    - aware of her need for rest
    - aware of her hunger and fullness cues.

Guiding somatic movements using language that emphasizes the enjoyment of movement for its own sake rather than to fix or improve anything, perhaps peppered with the positive qualities of adipose tissue, may help a woman inhabit her body less judgmentally and with more pleasure.

Later, offering self-led, improvised movement can boost self-esteem, as it may help a woman recognize that she has choice regarding her experience of her body, and does not need to listen to the external cues that may create body dissatisfaction. *I am large and the world says this should make me achy and graceless* may eventually transform into *I love to move my body this way.*

We don't need to suggest that a woman should love her body. In fact, more realistic, logical, and in keeping with yoga, is to feel neutral about it. It's a body. It is fascinatingly incredible, but also mundanely functional, as all bodies are. It eats and poops! But to love the feel of it moving, or the whisper of a breeze on the skin, or the burst of flavor of a mindfully eaten apple … oh my! That is available to all humans if we can tune in to the body's true experiences rather than hating or indeed idolizing it …

Libido changes

Usually listed as "loss of libido", I prefer to talk about libido changes. This is because it's not always about decreased libido, but also because using the word "loss" may front-load a woman's experience. Perhaps some women don't see it as a loss … Nevertheless, many women find reduced libido a troubling symptom of perimenopause.

It makes absolute biological sense that libido reduces when reproductive capability reduces. Unfortunately, society tells us that we should continue to be fabulously sexual forever, and indeed sex can be the glue that holds valued relationships together.

Some women, however, experience increased libido, and some of them find that that includes noticing a desire for a change of partner. We don't know why. More than one factor may be contributing. For instance, the MT is a time when many women begin to question their lives in every aspect. What am I here for? What do I want from life?

Increased libido may possibly be due to decrease in estrogen leading to more unopposed testosterone, or possibly to an *increased* body confidence—not the most common tendency, but not as unusual as you might expect during the body's last attempt to conceive. This is not just about confidence in appearance, but sexual confidence, knowing what she wants, and being more in control of her own pleasure during sex.

Things we have allowed to go under the radar, or we have put up with, become more obvious sources of unease, like an overly stressful or unsatisfying job, partnership, diet, exercise regime, or friendship. If we find ourselves unable to ignore a disappointment in, or lack of passion for, an intimate relationship, that may of course affect libido.

However, if a woman is in the last months of her possible reproductive capability, it would be logical that her libido might rise, and in her search for a mate, she looks for the strongest specimen, and so perhaps finds herself looking elsewhere. Many women I have worked with one-on-one, who have committed relationships, speak about attraction to possible sexual partners outside their relationship and/or feeling that they are frustrated by or feel less love for their partner. They harbor shame around this. Understanding the biochemistry and anthropology of menopause may help a woman be less hard on herself, and may help her figure out whether her changing satisfaction with her mate is because change is overdue, or whether it is a passing phase brought about by fluctuating hormones that will settle.

Coming back to the issue of *reduced* libido, even if a woman accepts it as normal, and doesn't miss it, even if she doesn't desire sex, how can she avoid the potential relationship wounds that may occur? And what if, for her, pleasure means sex, and sex means pleasure? How can she find pleasure in her body, and joy in her life?

What you can offer

Good news for teachers: a study in 2009 found that yoga helped with sexual function, satisfaction, and orgasm in a cohort of women doing yoga, and helped especially the women aged between 45 and 55. There was no control group, so more research is needed, but these women reported improvements over a 12-week yoga practice (Dhikav et al, 2010). In general, all the pleasure and somatic practices you read about earlier, and the attention to what feels pleasant in the body or her environment which I detailed when speaking about Organic Intelligence practices, are rich resources for you as a teacher, as is the movement meditation at the end of p.152.

Outside of yoga

Before addressing libido, help your student remember that pleasure is still available and can and should be sought. Avenues for this are in Chapter 3 c).

Suggest she consider her attitude toward this change and toward her body. Her relationship with her body and the world is changing, and the only way to manage change healthily and sustainably is to accept and adapt to it.

I spoke to relationship and sexuality counselor Fiona Daly, and these are the incredibly valuable insights she offered. Be aware, of course, that you do not need to heal every issue for your students, and we are not all qualified to offer advice on sexual or relationship matters. But some of these perspectives may help your student or her partner.

"Be aware that your sexual desire is unlikely to be completely gone. But the change from it being a central driving force can make it feel that way," Fiona says. If a woman tunes in, she may find that her libido is responding, but just more quietly. So she could listen attentively. "Think of it as an ember," says Fiona, "rather than a fire. Sometimes those embers will glow." These stirrings may be ones that she wouldn't have pursued in her twenties, but what happens if she listens when the whispers say, *I think I'd like to play?*

The nervous system will know if we are forcing things, and it will put the brakes on. As Fiona says, "Libido is a long game that the body will only play when it trusts you're not going to push it too far."

Why might women force things?
Fiona suggests some possibilities:

- Maybe her partner is expressing their loss or pressuring her.
- Maybe she has identified as a very sexual person and struggles with adapting to being a person for whom sex is taking a back seat.
- Maybe social media is telling her that her value is dependent on her sexual attractiveness and fabulousness in bed.

Perhaps there is still a glowing ember of desire. "Desire ignites through closeness," says Fiona, but maybe she's afraid to get close and is feeling a growing gulf?

Why would a woman be afraid to get close?
Apart from just not being in the mood, Fiona suggests that it might be because:

- she is concerned that if she approaches her partner with affection, it will be misread and she will feel pressure to have sex she doesn't want;
- she wants to be sensual but is afraid her body won't be able to follow through to the expected, climactic end-point of sexual activity;
- she thinks she would like sex but is afraid it will hurt.

What's advised in partnership?
Fiona says a woman needs to talk to her partner. She must tell them how she is feeling, physically, mentally, and emotionally. She might try saying:

- "Sometimes I want a little sensual affection, but I can't trust that I can see it through, so I don't approach you."
- "Can we find a way to be physical knowing that it doesn't inevitably have to include sex?"
- "Can I snuggle you with zero pressure?"
- "I feel a glow, but I'm scared that if I begin, the ember will extinguish as soon as something starts. If I know you understand that, then I will feel more free."

It strikes me that if women begin to get affectionate again with a partner initially in circumstances where it can't move on to sex, that could take the pressure off: snuggling on a park bench, arm in arm on a walk, holding hands in a café. Because our nervous system is the boss. The safer we feel, the more our body softens toward permission and pleasure.

So, it may be a matter of a woman being patient with herself, understanding that her body is changed, and that it truly is okay not to be a sexual goddess, accepting that she needs more patience and care, but also that intimacy, even sexual intimacy, doesn't need to have a beginning, a middle, and an end, and it certainly shouldn't be painful.

We have a lifetime of programming from the movies, telling us what sex should be, what constitutes a worthwhile old age, and what denotes a successful relationship. Perhaps women could take time to reconstruct their own physical future, beginning with their instinct as to what they *truly* want and need now. It will forever change. She may be able to help herself, and her partner if she has one, to change with it, so that she can meet her true self at every valuable moment of her life.

B) PROTECTING HEALTH

In this section I offer you an overview of some key systems in our bodies, why they are significant, and how we can support them in general, through yoga, and through nutrition.

Digestive health
The changing biology
The hormone changes can deeply and negatively affect the gut. Digestion can be affected, with a slowing metabolism potentially slowing gut transit and creating constipation. Some women experience an increased incidence of reflux, and in later life the digestive system can become less efficient at absorbing all the nutrients we need.

Gut health and the microbiome are also big players in the way we process MHT and phytoestrogens. The gut and the liver are central to our ability to process and excrete any toxins, whether from medications, from food or from hormones created in abundance in our bodies (which can be the case in the LRS and early perimenopause, when estrogen can sometimes surge). Once the liver has done its job, we need regular bowel motions to excrete those toxins.

How yoga can help
You may think digestive health is not in your gift to solve, but given that stress is one of the most significant factors affecting gut health, you have many supportive tools at your fingertips.

The gut is connected to the brain via the conversation of the amygdala with the vagus nerve. The vagus nerve affects mood. The sympathetic nervous system, when activated, shuts down digestion, which can lead to acute and chronic digestive issues.

You can certainly share tips on mindful eating. As well as helping with absorption, mindful eating may reduce bloating and reflux. It may even add pleasure to our eating experience! How? Try taking three breaths before eating, eating in a calm environment, eating away from screens and work, chewing very well and eating slowly, and you may notice you appreciate your food more, and thereby are satiated more easily. In addition, eating without distractions allows for better nutrient absorption, and eating in itself helps stimulate the feel-good hormones. A triple whammy of feel-good benefit!

Here I offer you two more physical paths to gut and vagus nerve health.

Abdominal massage

This is a self-administered version of the abdominal part of Thai massage. As taught in the practical hours of my teacher training course, always massage clockwise and suggest your client be led by what feels good on a given day. Avoid painful pressure.

1) Lying on your back, or standing up if that's not possible, place your hands on your belly and begin to stroke in a clockwise direction, with whatever pressure feels good. Continue for a minute or so.

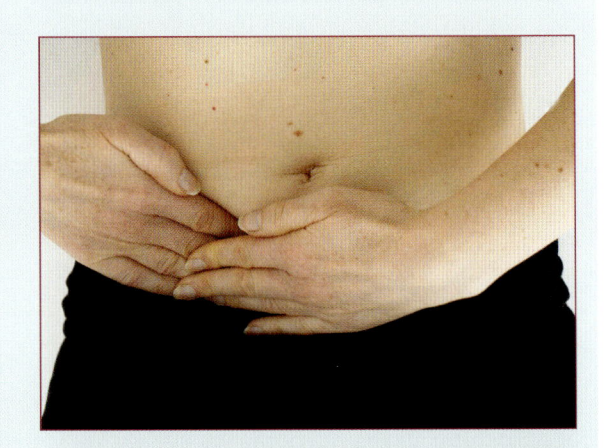

2) Beginning at the lower right quadrant, press the four fingers of one hand (with the other on top if you desire) gently into the abdomen and gently circle them.

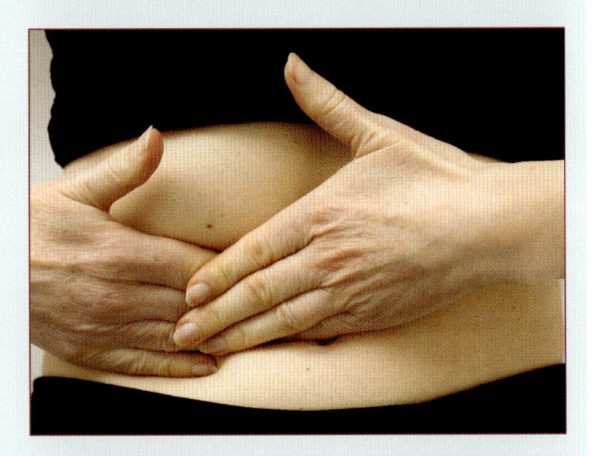

3) Imagining a clock-face, do this all around the belly at approximately each of the five-minute points.

    Stroke lightly again for a minute.

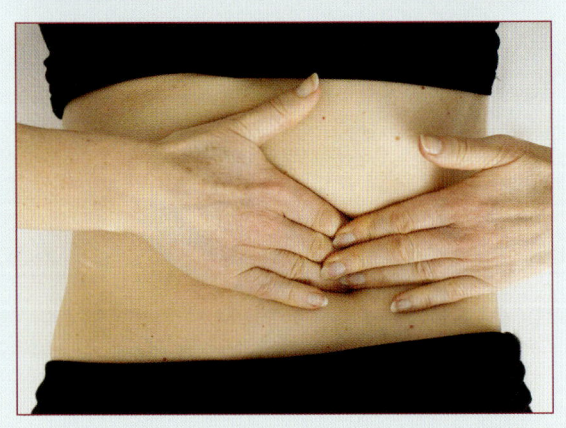

4) Then, imagining your belly as the 6 side of a dice, with two thumbs press gently but deeply into two dots either side of the lower belly. Take a breath or two, allowing the inhale to push the thumbs out, then depress them on the exhale.

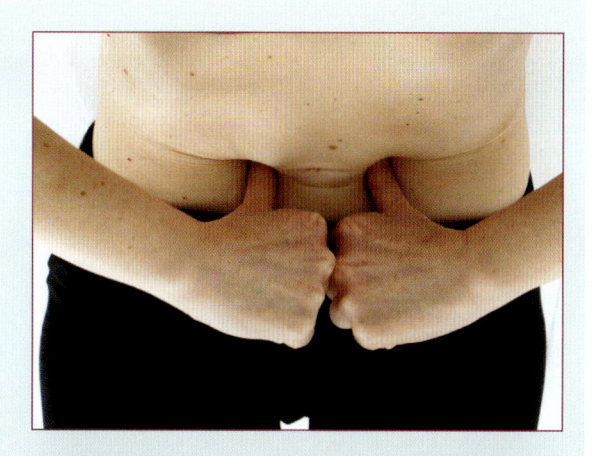

5) Move up the dice to two points on each side of the navel, about an inch or two away from it. Use the same breath and pressure as above.

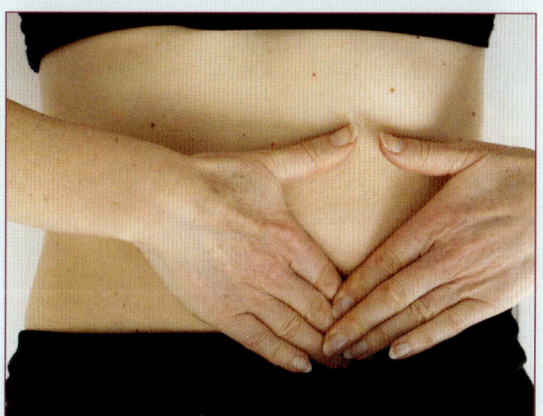

6) Move the thumbs up to the next points of the dice (upper abdomen) and repeat. Spend some time with the stroking motion again. Rest.

You can add your own techniques if you have massage experience.

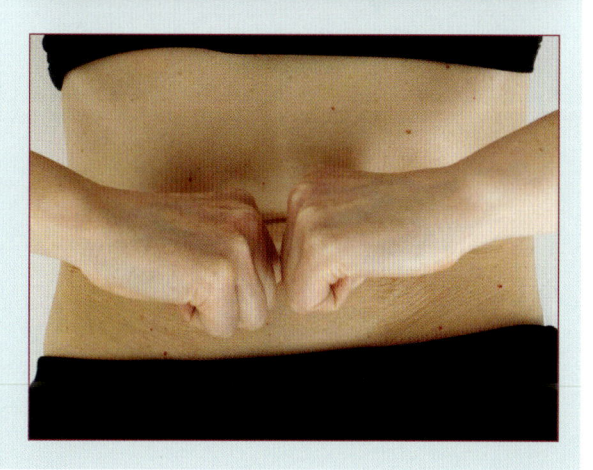

Movement
Twists, backbends, and bent-knee forward folds may help with the gut and vagus nerve, simply because the compression and release aid the flow of blood and lymph in the area, and they stimulate areas where the vagus nerve travels.

Please remember osteopenia/osteoporosis contraindications clarified in Chapter 4 a) on p.112–115, regarding twists and forward folds.

Uddiyana bandha and kaphalabhati may also be a valuable tools as they stimulate the abdomen.

Help outside yoga
Nutrition
The easiest nutrition tip to take away with you in relation to gut health is variety. You may have heard of the recommendation doing the rounds to eat 30 different plant foods per week. That doesn't mean full portions of 30 different plant foods a week, just 30 species! And it's not just vegetables. Spices and grains, pulses, and even different colors of the same vegetable, like peppers and onions, count toward variety too.

This is in part a recommendation for gut health. Bacteria are essential for gut health, and each strain of bacteria needs to eat. What they eat is fiber and each likes different food. Hence, we aim to give them what they demand by our varied intake.

Fiber-rich plant foods (containing prebiotics) to choose from: whole grains, vegetables, seeds, garlic, onions, artichoke, inulin, psyllium husks.

Fermented foods (containing probiotics) help to bolster the bacteria in the gut. They include tempeh, kimchi, sauerkraut, kombucha. Live foods like yogurt and kefir do a similar job.

Motility
Bowel movements are important for detoxification, but they can become less reliable as the decades go by, which can have an impact on the comfort and health of later life, so maintaining a regular bowel habit is a vital consideration.

The consumption of both soluble and insoluble fibers is essential for motility. Insoluble fibers are abundant in the husks and skins of plant foods. Soluble fibers are mostly found inside the plant: the flesh of an apple, sweet potato, or bean, for example.

Hydration is extremely important too. Don't increase fiber without increasing hydration, and don't increase it suddenly, but in small increments.

Foods that aid motility include apples and pears (which contain pectin), ginger, beetroot, dried fruit, green leafy vegetables (high in magnesium, known to help relieve constipation), papaya, soaked chia and flax seeds, and husks.

Absorption
Some digestive issues occur because of a reduction in the production of digestive enzymes. This can make for uncomfortable

symptoms, but also, in later life, lead to inefficient absorption of essential nutrients. How can we help the production of those enzymes?

- Cooking—and looking at—your meal
- Chewing bitter foods like arugula (rocket)
- Eating slowly and chewing well
- Consuming bone broth (contains glutamine which supports the immune system, the brain, and digestion)
- Taking peppermint tea or supplement (relaxes gut wall)
- Including sauerkraut in your diet.

How you eat is as important as what you eat. Remember mindful eating.

If you suffer from digestive issues, it may be worth keeping a diary of what you eat and removing any foods that you identify as possible triggers. At the same time, increase foods with anti-inflammatory properties (listed on p.185). Specifically for digestion, peppermint and bone-broth can be soothing.

The liver
The changing biology
The liver is the "gatekeeper" of our health, like a bouncer at a nightclub: nothing that circulates in your bloodstream gets there without the approval of your liver (figure 5.1). It will cast out any riff-raff! But a high number of riff-raff can take their toll. It is burdened by everything to which our organism is exposed.

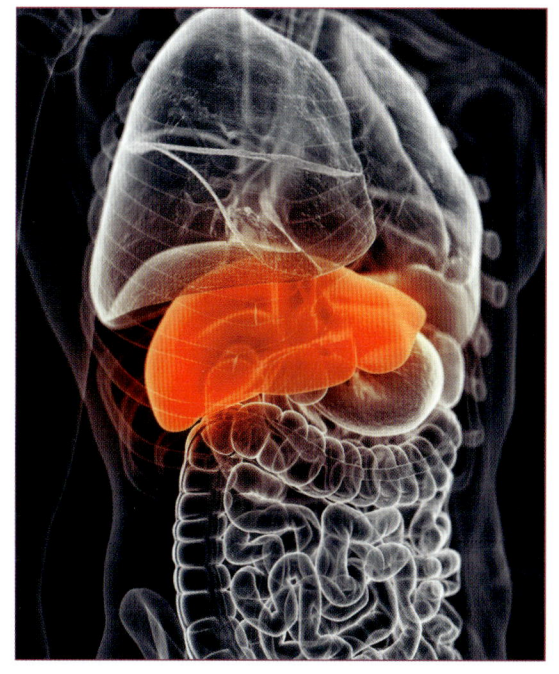

Figure 5.1 *Our liver is big! Damage has major implications but it can regenerate really well*

The liver is so important that evolution has made it the only organ that can regenerate. Considered part of the digestive system, it performs over 500 functions for the smooth running of the human body, and supporting liver health is important for them all. In addition to converting toxins and used hormones so that they can be excreted, the liver has wider essential functions:

- It produces bile, which is essential in breaking down cholesterol and aiding the digestion of fats, proteins, and some vitamins.
- It stores up to a year's worth of vitamin supplies.

- It metabolizes our carbohydrate intake to release glucose into the bloodstream to keep energy levels stable (keeping an extra store on hand for moments of sudden requirement).
- It has immune-supportive capability.
- It supports blood-pressure and blood-vessel integrity.
- It manufactures cholesterol, which is the building block for some of our hormones, such as estrogen, progesterone, and cortisol.
- It produces IGF-1, which stimulates growth, especially of the bones.
- And perhaps most importantly for our study, research shows that how the liver responds to estrogen is linked to our metabolism and our immunity, especially after menopause (Della Torre et al, 2011).

Look again at that list. Do you see how relevant it is to menopause?

In early perimenopause it has to deal with higher levels of estrogen, and later with higher levels of cortisol and cholesterol. In addition, it can become more sluggish.

Some early signs of a struggling liver:

- fatigue
- general malaise
- nausea
- loss of appetite
- tenderness in liver area
- disturbed sleep
- spidery red capillaries on upper abdomen
- pale stool
- difficulty digesting fats.

The most common liver problems caused by lifestyle are alcohol-related liver disease (ARLD) and non-alcoholic fatty liver disease (NAFLD), which can lead to cirrhosis (fibrosis, leading to non-functioning of liver tissue). We can lessen the likelihood of NAFLD by keeping fructose and other refined sugars to a minimum. Caring for blood sugar stability may help avoid insulin resistance, which is a risk factor for NAFLD.

How yoga can help

Please remember that you have neither the responsibility to heal anyone's liver, nor, unless otherwise qualified, the skills to do so. But …

- Movement is key to liver health, so … teach asana!
- If you are interested in traditional Chinese medicine, stimulate the liver meridian (inner thighs).
- Aerobic and resistance training are liver-supportive, so use the bone and muscle strength techniques we have learned. Recommend hiking, dancing, etc., for aerobic health.

Help outside yoga
Nutrition

Here's a quick rundown.

- Increase levels of omega-3 (the good fats) to help reduce inflammation, fat accumulation, and NAFLD. These are most efficiently found in oily fish like **s**ardines, **m**ackerel, **a**nchovies, **s**almon, **h**erring, and **t**rout (SMASHT), but also are in nuts, seeds, avocado, olive oil, and flax oil.

- Include antioxidants to balance free radicals and inflammation (see p. 185).
- There are detoxifiers, or more accurately, substances that support the production of enzymes that detoxify. They are found in beetroot, blueberries, and cruciferous vegetables. NB: The liver needs protein to function, so juice-only "detox" regimes may not be liver-supportive.
- Foods rich in anti-inflammatory compounds may help to reduce fibrosis and scar tissue (see p.185–186).
- The following may support bile production: bitter foods (arugula/rocket, chicory, curly salad), dandelion leaf, artichoke, beetroot, coffee. Make sure the bitterness is detectable, because it is the taste that gets those enzymes flowing.
- Hydrate.

Protection

Here is a brief list of some additions and subtractions that are widely recommended as supportive for liver health:

- Regulation of blood sugar
- Aerobic exercise
- Resistance training
- Stabilizing weight: However, larger active people have reduced liver fat compared with larger sedentary people, meaning we can improve liver health without weight loss (Stine et al, 2023)
- Checking with a doctor before adding supplements to the diet if using medication
- Avoiding or reducing alcohol intake (maximum two drinks at any one time)
- Avoiding recreational drugs
- Avoiding chemical-laden cosmetics and cleaning products
- Considering vaccines if traveling to countries where malaria and hepatitis are common.

Heart health
The changing biology

Postmenopause, women's previously lower risk of heart disease matches that of men. Finally, equality! But to be serious, in Chapter 1 you read some of the reasons why. Cardiovascular (CV) health needs to be taken seriously by women in a way that they may have not come to expect, being perhaps culturally more inclined to consider breast and cervical health.

How yoga can help

Yoga already supports heart health, and we can enhance that. As always, though there are so many areas to care for, remember that everything we do to care for any system will have a positive impact on others.

- Exercise supports good cholesterol levels, so continue to offer asana.
- Movement will support vascular tissue, and you can be more specific by adding movement in the heart area with some arm-swinging in your warm-ups (enhancing mood at the same time). This will also increase heart rate.
- Muscle mass and demand affect CV health, so focusing more on strength in asana is good for the heart. Add those bone-friendly resistance bands if you feel comfortable to do so.
- Inflammation impacts the heart, so anything you do to ease stress and inflammation will support the heart,

and stress reduction will support blood pressure. So keep offering de-stress takeaway practices to relieve anxiety and aid sleep along the way. Pepper effort and rest, effort and rest through your classes.
- Yoga can contribute to balancing blood sugars.
- Breathing deeply, including pranayama, supports your lungs and heart. So your pelvic floor health breathing practices are also a sneaky heart support! The list goes on—a biotensegrity.

Help outside yoga

Recommend activities that increase heart rate, like a walk where a woman speeds up for a few minutes every now and then, or walks fast up any small hill that's on her route, and slows down again after a bit, or swimming laps, which also moves the arms a lot, meaning that the heart will be physically moving.

Nutrition

Brain and heart health are intimately linked, so you might want to remind yourself of the nutrition section for the brain in Chapter 4. As well as tying in with the brain, CV health is greatly affected by systemic inflammation and blood sugar regulation. So all the tips on looking after these elements in this chapter would be included in heart-healthy eating.

More specifically for the heart:

- Salt is essential for life, so never give up salt completely, but for the sake of blood pressure, salt intake should be kept lower than in the menstrual years.
- Wholegrain products have been seen to reduce risks to heart health, where refined versions increase risk.
- Magnesium is particularly important for the heart (along with all the other micronutrients). It is found in abundance in green leafy vegetables, which also contain artery-protective vitamin K.
- Nuts and seeds are abundant sources of micronutrients and of fibers, which have a role to play in cholesterol regulation.
- Garlic and the onion family contain a compound called allicin, beneficial for blood-sugar, blood pressure and cholesterol levels.
- Here are a few tips for supporting cholesterol balance:
  - Reduce, but do not omit, saturated fats.
  - Reduce sugar and alcohol.
  - Increase soluble and insoluble fiber, increasing fluids at the same time.
  - Consider supplementing fiber with psyllium husks. It would be wise to seek guidance from a functional medicine practitioner/nutrition therapist. If you're confident, go slow: start with a teaspoon a day in a glass of water, and increase over weeks to perhaps 3 tsp per day. Stop if there is bloating or discomfort.
  - Increase omega-3 fats.
  - Consider supplementing with plant sterols. Start with a low dose, and check with your doctor first.
  - Stop smoking.
  - Avoid overeating, particularly near bedtime.

Systemic inflammation
The changing biology
I wrote about this on p.171–172. Have a look back to remind yourself of the changes in our inflammation response that impacts women physically, but also significantly impacts cardiovascular, brain, and gut health.

So managing inflammation can impact health positively and widely. Further effects of slightly or more considerably elevated inflammation can include fibromyalgia, leaky gut, chronic fatigue, and more. The symptoms of these overlap with some symptoms of perimenopause.

How you can help
We can point out some of the suggestions on general inflammation discussed in the section on aching joints, recommending perhaps massage and/or physiotherapy (or the doctor) to check for any structural issues.

Movement and massage are positive interventions for managing inflammation because they stimulate and support the lymphatic system, which is one of the key regulators of the inflammation response.

Continuing to engage in any practices that support the vagus nerve and help to regulate stress is also of value.

Help outside yoga
Nutrition
Some eating patterns can contribute to inflammation. People with diets low in whole grains, fruits, and vegetables may be more likely to experience inflammation. A woman may have old or newly developed sensitivities that they could have investigated.

I would recommend that a woman with chronic inflammation and/or digestive issues should see a nutrition professional to investigate potential triggers. We should avoid suggesting elimination diets without professional support.

Some foods with possible anti-inflammatory properties: whole grains, alliums like garlic and onion, turmeric, berries, oily fish, cherries, tomatoes, nuts, fermented foods, green vegetables, beetroot, fruit, beans, cocoa, green tea, and coffee.

Dietary patterns that may contribute to inflammation: consuming a lot of trans-fats, refined carbohydrates, sugar, red meat (in particular, processed meat), gluten (only if you are sensitive), refined oils, processed foods, and saturated fats.

Fighting free radicals
Reducing free-radical damage and oxidative stress can help to reduce chronic inflammation by reducing damage to healthy cells. To do this:

- Avoid cooking with light seed oils.
- Cook with olive oil for shorter times at lower temperatures, and ghee or coconut oil at higher temperatures or for longer.
- Reduce alcohol and stop smoking.
- Have gaps of at least a couple of hours between eating.
- Keep hydrated.

- Antioxidants play a part in the fight against free radicals, so when enjoying any foods that may have more free radicals, like charred foods from the barbeque, add some antioxidant-rich food like a salad.
- Over the course of a day, especially if you are enjoying fast foods like pizza or shop-bought biscuits/cakes, ensure you have antioxidant-rich foods that day too. Antioxidants are found in abundance in most vegetables and fruit, in particular, berries, leafy greens, artichoke, beetroot, and nuts and beans. Dark chocolate is rich in antioxidants too.

The lymphatic system
The changing biology

The lymphatic system is central to our wellbeing, and dysregulations therein can cause clear and more subtle issues, including systemic inflammation (figure 5.2). It is the system which supports our immune system, as lymph is replete with a variety of disease-fighting cells. In addition, it is like a water-treatment plant, filtering waste, bacteria, damaged and rogue cells that leech by osmosis from our blood to our tissues. Lymph collects tissue fluids and filters them at the lymph nodes, before returning these fluids to the blood for eventual excretion via the usual excretory channels. Further, it helps with the absorption of fats and fat-soluble vitamins from our digestive system, enabling their use as fuel, and maintains fluid balance in the body.

Disorders can include lymphedema, characterized by swelling, mostly of the limbs, though it can occur in the chest, neck, belly, and groins, and can develop into stiffness and further symptoms. It can be caused by radiation treatment, surgical removal of lymph nodes, and by cancerous growths themselves.

There is ongoing research into the effects of estrogen on the lymphatic system as lymphedema post-cancer can develop years later, suggesting a possible correlation between estrogen-blocking medications (required after some cancers) and lymphedema, rather than the immediate cancer treatment (Garmy-Susini, 2019).

This effect of changing estrogen because of medication suggests that menopause *may* have an effect on the efficient functioning of the lymphatic system, so it warrants attention. Possible symptoms of non-optimal lymphatic function, such as bloating, swelling, weight gain, headaches, joint pain, and fatigue, are common among women in perimenopause.

Before we get into supporting the lymphatic system through yoga, we must note: **Any gut and/or limb swelling should be checked by a doctor.**

How yoga can help

We know that the lymphatic system has no pump and that muscular contraction and gravity are what it relies on to keep moving. Therefore yoga may be a very valuable resource for its care. Learning the sites of the major players in the lymphatic system can help you as a teacher to choose key areas to address through movement.

A JOURNEY, SUPPORTED 187

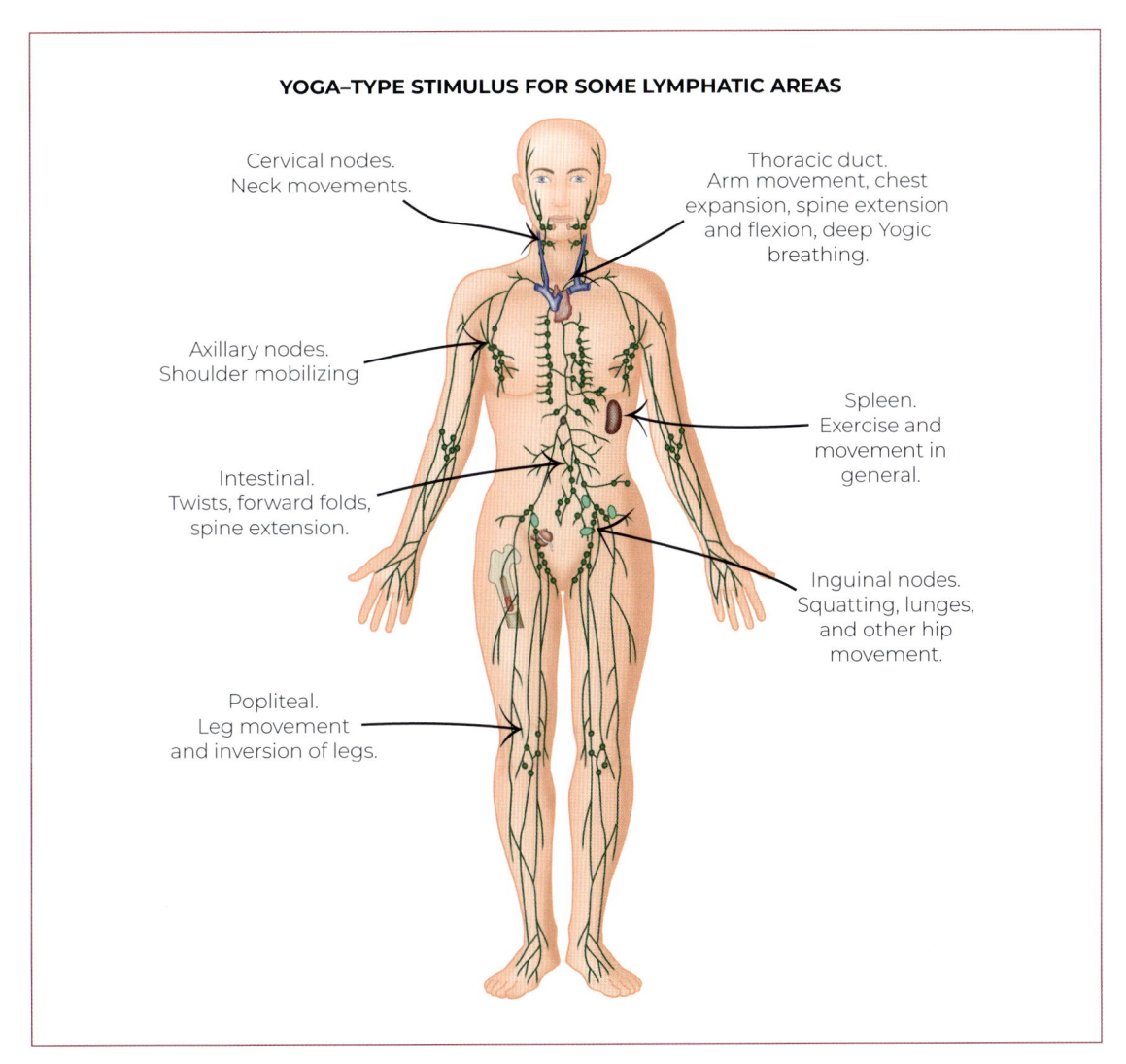

YOGA–TYPE STIMULUS FOR SOME LYMPHATIC AREAS

- Cervical nodes. Neck movements.
- Thoracic duct. Arm movement, chest expansion, spine extension and flexion, deep Yogic breathing.
- Axillary nodes. Shoulder mobilizing
- Spleen. Exercise and movement in general.
- Intestinal. Twists, forward folds, spine extension.
- Inguinal nodes. Squatting, lunges, and other hip movement.
- Popliteal. Leg movement and inversion of legs.

Figure 5.2 *Lymphatic system*

Anyone with lymphedema should be addressing this through expert care only. Please remind yourself of contraindications including congestive heart failure, history of clots and/or stroke, liver and/or kidney issues, and current infection.

Self-touch for lymphatic support

Some of these areas are easy to self-massage appropriately, but though simple, this is not in my gift to teach. However, touch stimulus can be suggested for healthy individuals. Keep in your awareness: direction (toward the heart), pressure (light), and pace (slow). You may choose to suggest a few techniques for self-care through touch:

- Light, downward, pulsing stretch of the skin of the side of the neck
- Gentle pressure just above collar bones

- Scooping skin of the armpit from arm to trunk (just enough to move the skin surface)
- Stroking of hands on the groins in the direction of the navel.

Movement stimulus

As well as light touch, movement is key for the lymphatic system to function. Any movement is beneficial, but we can target movement in areas with an abundance of lymph nodes.

From standing or sitting:

- Any neck movement
- Shoulder scrunching and releasing
- One hand behind the head, raise and lower the elbow
- Interlace hands behind back
- Standing forward fold.

Other positions:

- Downward dog
- Legs up the wall
- Squatting
- Bridge pose
- Twists.

Also the movement associated with diaphragmatic breathing and uddiyana bandha will stimulate key areas also.

Help outside yoga

Outside of yoga, we can look after our lymphatic system by reducing toxic exposure much the same as for the liver—by hydrating with water, by deep breathing, eating a healthy diet, reducing stress, and by moving. Lymphatic massage could be suggested, but note that it is contraindicated for people with congestive heart failure, history of clots and/or stroke, liver and/or kidney issues, and current infection.

Blood sugar regulation
The changing biology

Perimenopause can make it harder to regulate optimal levels of blood sugar. This has immediate symptomatic effects and long-term health impacts. Avoiding blood-glucose peaks and troughs may be the easiest and most far-reaching adjustment you can make for many perimenopausal symptoms, and for your future health.

The effects of unstable blood sugar may help you see why this is an important area to be looking after in perimenopause. They include:

- Sleep disturbance
- Anxiety
- High cortisol
- Hot flashes
- Difficulty concentrating
- Carbohydrate craving.

Long-term high blood sugar can lead to insulin resistance, implicated in many diseases associated with aging. Insulin resistance causes the body to be unable to metabolize blood glucose and can lead on to type 2 diabetes. The risk of developing it is higher in perimenopause and beyond.

Balanced blood sugars may support:

- Consistent energy
- Less cortisol
- More stable mood

- Feeling of satiety
- Cognitive function
- Improved metabolism
- Reduced inflammation
- Better heart, brain, and bone health.

How yoga can help
There is convincing evidence that yoga can help prevent pre-diabetes progressing to type 2 diabetes. This is good news!

Help outside yoga
Exercise is beneficial. Not just big exercise, but even housework or walking the dog is beneficial, even just for a short time, and especially soon after eating. This has been seen to help with blood-sugar regulation. Knowing this information eased my resentment around tidying the kitchen after dinner instead of heading straight for the sofa! It also helped me feel okay about teaching a class soon after dinner, despite yoga's tradition of practicing on an empty stomach …

Other ways to balance blood sugar may give us some insight into why yoga seems to help:

- Rest
- Sleep
- Stress reduction.

Nutrition
Not eating regularly and not eating sufficient and *balanced* meals and snacks destabilizes blood sugar. A balanced meal or snack consists of three "macronutrients": protein, complex carbohydrate, and good fats. A complex carbohydrate is essentially one that contains fiber, such as whole grains and carb-rich vegetables. They are made up of many molecules strung together which means they take longer to break down into the molecules that can be absorbed into the bloodstream (glucose or fructose). Simple carbohydrates are just two molecules strung together, so the speed of digestion and assimilation is quicker, causing those blood-sugar spikes.

A macro balanced snack might be hummus on an oatcake, a little dark chocolate with a few nuts, or an apple with nut butter. Apples contain carbohydrate, including fiber, and the nuts have complex carbs, protein, and good fats. The apple alone lacks protein or good fat.

A macro balanced meal would be, for example, sardines on wholemeal toast, or chicken, cashew nut and vegetable stir-fry with brown rice.

We need micronutrients as well as macro. Micronutrients are the ones we can't see. Essentially you could think of them as the vitamins and minerals. So, for a more micronutrient-rich meal you would add a yummy salad to that sardines on toast option.

Overwhelmed?!

Remember that everything we do to support any one area of the body and its systems will support every other one!

CHAPTER 6
FOOD AND MEDICINE

NUTRITION

Diet and dieting

In general, when the body is undergoing any challenge, robust and varied nutrition is immensely important. Unfortunately, at perimenopause many women reduce their nutritional intake in a bid to avoid the changes they see to their shape and composition.

> **Please do not use anything I say here about nutrition for more than just your own information, unless you have a qualification in nutrition.**
>
> In training as a nutrition coach, we learn that recommending supplements in a group setting is *not* responsible because they can have interactions with medications participants may be taking, or be problematic with certain health issues. In these cases, the use of supplements should be checked with a doctor. So I am not covering them here.

We know that eating too little usually means not meeting our basic micronutrient needs (Calton, 2010) or, of course, our energy needs. In addition, calorie deficit dieting can increase the risk of osteoporosis. Carbohydrate restriction in diets like Keto can have the same effect (Fensham et al, 2022; Simm et al, 2017; Heikura et al, 2020), and indeed the Keto diet has been seen to cause constipation (Wibisono et al, 2015), possibly because of a lack of fiber. Keto, though it can improve fasting blood sugars, may be dangerous for people with type 1 diabetes (Leow et al, 2018) and though intermittent fasting has some positive results, at least in the short term (Coyle, 2018), it and other controlled ways of eating can increase the risk of developing eating disorders (Colombarolli et al, 2022; Grave, 2020).

Ensuring she gives her body adequate food may not only help to avoid the above risks, but also result in greater and more consistent energy, less joint pain, better sleep, a greater sense of happiness, better concentration, and less inflammation.

Our whole body is interrelated, so that, for instance, adequate nutrition without addressing digestive issues may not be the best way to holistically support health and energy. Lifting weights without adequate nutrition is to try to build bone with too few raw materials. Doing brain-training exercises without sufficient fuel for the brain may be to waste your time.

Emotional eating

Currently we are told that "emotional eating" is bad, but consider a baby; what does it first turn to in order to feel safe? The breast. Consider sitting down to eat with people you love whom you haven't seen for a long time. Is that only macro and micro nutrition you are experiencing or does it nourish you in other ways? Consider eating a food you associate with a happy time in your youth. Is it bad if that makes you feel closer to long-lost loved ones, or if it makes you weep with the intensity of the nostalgia?

We might benefit from remembering that eating is emotional from birth. We have different types of hunger, which all deserve attention. Food is not just nutrition but also community and pleasure. It can stimulate the brain to produce the endorphins that bring us a sense of wellbeing.

But if there is a struggle with disinhibited eating one might make these suggestions:

- Try to pause ... Listen to the urge ... Ask "What kind of hunger is this?" (taste, energy, comfort).
- If it's comfort, ask "What are my needs?"
- Ask "How else might I meet them?" (call a confidante, climb under a blanket, get out in the air, find someone for a hug, watch a weepy movie to release some tears, yell, walk, read a book with a cup of tea).
- Ask "Am I tired?" If yes, then rest first (10–20 minutes lying down/restorative pose, eyes closed) then tune in again to hunger if it's still there.
- Ask "Am I thirsty?" If yes, drink first, then tune in again to hunger if it's there.
- If hunger is still there, ask "Do I want something ... savory, sweet, hot, cold, crunchy, smooth, etc.?"
- Ask "What's available?"

Then take your time. Choose your favorite crockery. Sit. Indulge with pleasure.

Remember, you can't eat your way out of tiredness if your body needs rest, and you can't rest yourself to regain energy if your body or brain need food.

Phytoestrogens

When writing about nutrition and menopause there must be a mention of phytoestrogens. These are compounds naturally occurring in plant species which have estrogen-like qualities and can mimic estrogen when present in the body. They are widely touted as promoting health and relieving perimenopausal symptoms. Many women find them very beneficial.

There is some evidence to support the consumption of foods rich in phytoestrogens to reduce hot flashes (Chen et al, 2020) and even improve bone health. Most research currently confirms they are safe, but it would be essential to speak to your doctor before using phytoestrogen supplements. It seems always to be the case that consumption through foods is safer than consumption via supplements. A great article, 'Are Phytoestrogens Good for You?' (White & Cherney, 2021), contains links to relevant studies and is available online.

Most plants contain them, but below is a list of foods particularly rich in phytoestrogens which, after further research and advice from a nutrition professional and her doctor, a woman may choose to consume (or reduce, if she is concerned):

- Soya (edamame, miso tofu, etc.)
- Flax seeds (ground or their oils)
- Red clover
- Oats
- Lentils
- Legumes (peanuts, beans, peas)
- Apples
- Sweet potatoes
- Sesame seeds.

As you can see, there are some really fabulously nutritious foods in that list, so avoiding them would need to be for very robust reasons.

Nutrition for menopause condensed

I have gone into considerable detail in previous chapters. Here I aim to boil it down for you into some key things to consider:

- To meet our needs, a balanced day would include a satisfying amount of food at an approximate ratio of **50% vegetables** and some fruit, **25% lean protein, 25% complex carbohydrates,** with an extra slice of **good fats.**
- **Regular nutrition and balanced blood sugars** are better for energy and brain power than having big gaps between meals.
- **Carbohydrates** are a nutritious and important source of fiber, energy, vitamins and minerals much needed in perimenopause and beyond.
- A wide array of **plant foods of varying types and colors** offers a wide array of fibers, antioxidants, vitamins and minerals.
- Our **protein** intake needs to be increased.
- "Good" fats (**omega-3s** in particular) are particularly valuable.
- We need **minerals** such as calcium for our bones and tissue repair, and magnesium, which also supports bones, sleep, and can help reduce muscle cramps.
- **Vitamins D and K2** are essential to bring calcium to the bones.
- **Hydration** is **essential** for every single bit of us.
- **Go easy on alcohol, caffeine, and refined sugar** as they may affect sleep, hot flashes, and/or low mood and anxiety.
- **Eating enough** is non-negotiable.

What to eat, put simply

In my training as a nutrition coach, we were taught to keep things simple. So, in giving you the pared-down list in table 6.1, I hope it may help you understand how valuable it would be now to let go of the whys.

Table 6.1 *What to eat, put simply*

A Quick Guide

- Plant food variety (30 per week)
- Protein (plenty and various)
- Calcium-rich foods dotted throughout the day
- Viamins D and K2
- Oily fish
- Nuts and seeds
- Olive oil
- Wholegrains
- Berries
- Beans and pulses
- Green leafy and cruciferous vegetables and beets
- Deeply colored foods (eat the rainbow)
- Fermented and live foods
- Hydration
- Macro-balanced meals and snacks
- Green tea, coffee, dark chocolate (in moderation)
- Eat slowly and stress-free

Making changes can begin by introducing a few foods every now and then until it becomes an almost effortless habit ...

MENOPAUSE HORMONE THERAPY

Please do not use this section for more than just your own information, unless you are medically qualified.

For many years menopause hormone therapy (MHT), also known as hormone replacement therapy (HRT) was feared, and yet now there are shortages of these medicines as it has become the first thing many women think of when they begin perimenopause. I have mentioned it a lot already. Now, let's go into a bit more detail about what we know, what we don't know, and the controversy that has come to surround it.

Thankfully, since compiling my course in early 2020, there have been huge changes in the visibility of menopause, and more women are talking about it freely. However, along with this we have a new burden: a polarization of women has become apparent.

Some women are passionately announcing their success stories through the use of MHT (or HRT), or diet or exercise practices. Those who have turned their experience around, and believe it is because of their chosen intervention, are sometimes harsh in their judgment of others' choices. As yoga teachers, we must remain open to all experiences, and modulate any damage caused by opinions being broadcast to or by our students.

This section has been fact-checked and reviewed by the esteemed consultant endocrinologist Dr Annice Mukherjee. She is instrumental in the bid to reduce the wild swing of the pendulum from the inflated narrative and promotion of MHT back to the more nuanced middle ground. If you are on social media, I recommend that you look at her work.

Part of this new drama is the result of some very important changes to what is accepted by the medical community. In 2002, the

Women's Health Initiative study into the risks of using MHT announced to the media that using it increased the risk of developing breast cancer. As a result, the use of MHT fell dramatically and doctors were afraid to prescribe it. More recently, it has come to light that the study was flawed and that the risks of MHT are much less than had been thought.

At present, there are some powerful voices advocating for its use even more unquestioningly (often on the basis of single studies) or at much higher doses than international guidelines recommend, and higher than are licensed on the basis of multiple studies. At the time of writing, for instance, a well-known private menopause doctor and her clinics are being scrutinized in the UK after it became clear that prescriptions at up to four times the licensed dosage were frequently being written, without this fact or the risk factors being made clear to the patients (Calman & Adams, 2023). The fact that this is happening is not disputed by the doctor in question. Indeed, it is not illegal to prescribe above the licensed dose. But the standard guidelines for MHT are clear: Start with the lowest possible dose, and when the top licensed dosage is reached, other interventions should be explored before increasing it further.

On a personal note, I was afraid to take MHT during my perimenopause because of that flawed study. I can't say for certain what I would have done if I knew then what I know now. I may have taken it for a few years, and if I had, perhaps I would not have such low bone density scores.

However, I know that I have several other risk factors for osteoporosis: family history, a small frame, and having been vegan for almost two decades. Symptomatically, I managed okay without MHT, thanks to my friends, my siblings, and to my interest in researching menopause and learning how to support myself.

I know many students who are taking MHT and thriving, many who are taking it and struggling. I know many who are not taking it and are thriving, many who are not taking it and are struggling. I am not anti-MHT; I know that it can protect certain areas of health, and I believe that, indirectly through alleviating devastating symptoms which may increase the risk of suicide in those struggling with depression or other mental health issues, it may save lives.

Here is what is known about MHT:

- It is the best intervention known for the relief of the symptoms of perimenopause.
- Taking MHT in perimenopause and early menopause can help to maintain bone strength.
- It is effective for the relief of genitourinary syndrome of menopause.
- Localized estrogen for the vagina appears to be extremely low risk due to the small dosage.
- MHT should first be offered at the lowest possible dose.
- MHT would be a recommended first line of intervention for protection of the health of those with premature/primary ovarian insufficiency (POI).

- At the time of writing, women are beginning to use testosterone, which has benefits for libido. Anecdotal reports of other benefits do not have any research backup as of January 2024.
- MHT is not recommended for chronic disease prevention.
- Women with a history or high risk of breast cancer or stroke are generally advised not to take it, or to use with very close supervision.
- Starting MHT more than ten years after your last period is associated with a higher level of health risks.
- Estrogen/progestogen (the synthetic form of progesterone) therapy seems to create more side effects and higher breast cancer risk than estrogen alone.
- Progestogens (or micronized progesterone, a more natural form) must be taken if a woman still has a womb.
- Transdermal estrogen administration seems to be safer than oral.
- Risk factors increase the longer you take it after natural menopause age and over 60 years of age. These risks include blood vessel disease, background breast cancer risk, and, with oral estrogens, an increased risk of deep vein thrombosis and stroke.
- Women should be prescribed on a case-by-case basis as one prescription does not fit all.
- Regular re-evaluation of treatment should be undertaken with risk factors discussed anew.
- Some women experience unpleasant side effects like nausea, bloating, breast tenderness or swelling, leg cramps headaches, bleeding, depression, and indigestion.
- MHT does not relieve every symptom; in particular anxiety, joint pain and brain fog may be difficult to alleviate.
- Lifestyle interventions to improve health outcomes are still important even when taking MHT, and may even increase its efficacy and your ability to tolerate it.

Research into the benefits of MHT to reduce Alzheimer's disease and dementia risk is ongoing. Some possible benefits, and some possible risks are still unclear. At the time of writing there have been some headlines regarding the results of a meta-analysis (Neratinni et al, 2023), one of whose authors, Dr Lisa Mosconi, is at pains to point out that though estrogen therapy may have some benefits, MHT is not approved for the purpose of preventing Alzheimer's disease. Once progestins or progestogens are added, the picture gets more complex in terms of risks.

Given that 80% of women **don't** develop Alzheimer's disease or dementia, and men also develop it, we cannot say that menopause causes it, so it makes sense that MHT is not going to be a definitive protection.

As much as they are sometimes given a bad rap, antidepressants can be effective for some symptoms where MHT is inappropriate or has been ineffective.

You can read more in these position statements from The Menopause

Society[4] (2022) and in the co-authored statement by respected bodies, including Dr Mukherjee and the British Menopause Society, the Royal College of Obstetricians and Gynaecologists, and the Society for Endocrinology listed in the bibliography (British Menopause Society, 2022).

Dr Mukherjee is one of the few realistic, balanced medical voices active on social media, and I offer you this content she published there. It offers an interesting perspective:

> *It is common to have a sense of relief when starting a new medication, especially when you've been led to believe it's needed. There can be a powerful placebo effect. So observational reports are not strong evidence. Placebo controlled trials eradicate reporting error.*
>
> *So if a benefit is not sustained, that is not a reason to increase your dose. It is a reason to re-evaluate and question efficacy.*
>
> *If your healthcare provider paints a picture about any treatment that seems too good to be true, it most probably is. Equally, if they dismiss any benefit of a treatment you were hoping to try, or have found beneficial, ask them to provide details of why they don't recommend it.*
>
> *Please don't second guess what you think future research may show. Evidence, not assumption, is fundamental to good healthcare. Otherwise information can be misconstrued and that can cause distress and harm.*[5]

YOUR RESPONSIBILITIES

It's worth reiterating for your protection and that of your students—although many symptoms of perimenopause are normal and passing and present no danger, it's possible for women to overlook a symptom of a disease and not attend for check-ups. Along with lots of other things which we should always bring to the doctor, we should not expect to manage such issues by healthy lifestyle alone, especially if improvements have been made to the four pillars of health but nothing is shifting.

As a teacher, you are not responsible for guessing what is going on in your students' bodies. But it may be helpful to you, if you become concerned, to keep in mind that, along with the usual "red flags" for any cohort, female or male, the following issues should be checked by a doctor.

- Unrelieved depression
- Unrelieved fatigue
- Symptoms that make it impossible to do everyday things
- Heavy bleeding that carries on for months
- Menstruating/bleeding *after* menopause
- Pelvic floor pain
- Unrelieved incontinence
- Bloating of limbs or abdomen
- Vaginal/vulval changes.

---

[4] Formerly the North American Menopause Society, which changed its name to The Menopause Society in July 2023, so your Google searches may be confusing!

[5] Annice Mukherjee, Instagram post, 2023.

AFTERWORD

IN SUMMARY

When you are working with women in midlife, and talking about menopause in your work, there may be more trust placed in you than you ask for, expect, or even warrant. There is no criticism here. I regularly find women expecting more of me than I can deliver. It's the beautiful nature of yoga teachers: we inspire trust. I believe that, to move closer to warranting that trust, we need to change the way we meet and teach all our students as *they* change, and to offer *ourselves* the same changing care.

Why should yoga change to accommodate menopause? I believe that:

- When the body becomes less able for strenuous and/or end-of-range-of-motion postures, women can lose confidence, self-esteem and a desire to continue their practice if alternatives are not adeptly delivered and demonstrated.
- Many of the various styles are slow to accept, or unaware of the need to make, changes in the way the resources of pranayama, meditation and asana are practiced.
- Due to physical changes, the expectation of constantly increasing flexibility may lead to greater risk of cartilage damage and/or arthritis
- In the West there is a considerable enmeshment of the world of yoga with diet culture, ageism, and the cult of the body-beautiful. Most yoga teachers feel a pressure to appear in their marketing, and in front of their students, as slim, bendy, and youthful. The result is that this is how most images of yoga appear. This is immensely impactful on a group of women who report hating the changes in their body, in particular weight, skin-tone, energy, and flexibility.
- The sense of yoga as a linear practice with a final goal in sight (the "full" expression of a pose, a regular meditation regime, competency in complex pranayama, daily practice, etc.) may make it damaging or difficult in the face of:
  - physical changes to tissues such as fascia, collagen, cartilage, and muscle
  - autonomic nervous system changes
  - symptoms like dizziness, fatigue, anxiety

- trauma resurgence
- time poverty
- typical family obligations at the average age of menopause.

I hope that in teaching *Yoga for Menopause and Beyond* you will prioritize:

- Yoga for the individual, rather than for the sake of yoga (acknowledging the variety of possible experiences)
- Community support (she is not alone)
- Sharing circles (to hear and be heard, a woman's experience is interesting and valued)
- Education (to push away fear and to empower)
- Perspectives (to open a woman's eyes to the effects of culture, ageism, and social pressures)
- Research (to make no baseless promises and to include reliable tools)
- Symptom care
- Avoidance of injury (nothing is worth risking injury when recovery can take longer and more severely impact quality of life)
- Stress reduction (in bite-sized achievable pieces available as triage and not just in class)
- Language adjustments (aware of and inclusive of all experiences and sensitivities)
- Instinctual movement (for self-agency, pleasure, and to move away from pain)
- Pleasure (for the release of feel-good hormones and to let go of pushing)
- Emotional exploration (for resiliency and self-acceptance)
- Science of stretch (to avoid injury and develop strength)
- Play (for relief from the seriousness of symptomatic struggles and fear)
- Self-determination (for self-esteem)
- Non-lineage approach (for empowerment and choice)
- Remembering some less frequently used tools from this great tradition (eye exercises for the brain, tongue exercises and chanting for the vagus nerve, the bandhas for strength)
- Supporting health concerns (my greatest passion now that I am postmenopausal!), especially
  - bones and muscles
  - pelvic floor
  - brain.

What would a yoga for menopause class look like?

If you wanted to tick every box in one session, it would be very long! Often this work is best done in a workshop format. But, after reading this book, you may find that all of your classes become, at the very least, "menopause friendly".

But if I was to be as brief and reductive as possible, a class might be:

- **Opening circle:** each woman has space to speak about struggles, symptoms, triumphs, questions.
- **Response:** teacher replies to this sharing with education, insights, tools, and perspective shifts.
- **Practice:**
  - **Breathing:** achievable breath practice with mention of evidence basis for its usefulness and suggestions as to how to take this into daily life for optimum benefit when not at yoga class.

- **Warm-up:** interoception-developing movement of your choice, like somatic-movement style practices, with improvisation suggested/allowed, pleasure mentioned as a possible focus. Indicate benefits of a little of this every day, in achievable circumstances.
- **Asana:** floor and/or standing strength-based asana reaching eustress, with added focus on muscle and bone stimulus, pelvic floor, balance, brain stimulus, functional flexibility, and injury avoidance. Offer strength or brain-training snacks students can perform during the week.
- **Relaxation:** extended relaxation, perhaps a restorative pose, plus shavasana, with touch offered.
- **Meditation:** guided meditation that addresses some common struggles, either at the end or during a restorative posture.

Throughout, I would expect a teacher to offer insights as to the evidence-based usefulness of the practices offered, what they support, and how a woman can add them to her week.

MY HOPES

For yoga and its teachers

In my dreams, one day the effects and changing needs of menopause, and how yoga can and should be adjusted to support it, will be taught as a matter of course in all yoga teacher trainings. Even entry-level short qualifications will have at least a page or two in the manual and devote a couple of hours to it at a minimum.

Taking a yoga for menopause further training will be as common as training in yoga for pregnancy, or even more so, because an average menopause has a bigger long-term impact on female health than an average pregnancy.

Just as with pregnancy, it behoves yoga teachers to understand the myriad issues that can arise, and what is advisable and not advisable for women whose hormones are changing, or have changed. So I hope this book, and others that will spring up, will empower teachers to know what they can and can't help with through yoga and how some common elements of yoga may be more damaging than supportive.

In addition to adjusting yoga to make it more menopause-supportive, I hope that in teachers and students we will see a development of deep acceptance for the perfections and struggles of the human organism, and respect for its needs at any life stage. I expect to see my trained teachers offer safety, self-acceptance, and a functional approach to the health and wellbeing of their students, perhaps in all their teaching, but in particular while teaching for the stages of menopause.

We are a maverick generation, researching, discovering, and speaking out to redress the imbalance which has seen this life-phase pushed into the periphery in the yoga world, as much as in the rest of the world.

I hope you will join me in aiming to soothe your students with the middle ground, with fact-based information and realistic hope, with no false promises and with a balanced, non-inflammatory attitude toward the possible impacts and ease of their perimenopause transition and the years beyond.

The women you are working with will be in and out of the peaks and troughs of the unpredictable variability of their hormonal changes for, on average, seven years. They will be more or less able to cope, and there will be many times when they think they are "through the other side". The knowledge you have taken the time to gain, and will pass on to them, will be invaluable to them. One phrase, one piece of information that you may consider insignificant or common knowledge, has the ability to devastate or to inspire, to confuse or to lift a veil.

I ask you to be gentle, to assume nothing, to acknowledge privately and publicly your abilities, and also your limitations, and to be sensitive to the hugely varying experiences and choices of the women you work with, or relate with in your community.

For women and for my daughters

If you had asked me my hopes back in 2020, I would have said that it was looking good: people were beginning to speak more freely; campaigners were making a difference through workplace talks and lobbying government to include menopause in education; science was re-thinking poorly-analyzed research on risks of MHT; and we were acknowledging and holding each other's struggles.

But asking me now, I am sadly less sure. Since 2021, and the release of a documentary on Channel 4 in the UK called *Sex, Myths and Menopause* which, though it created much-needed awareness and advocacy, sadly saw millions of women descend into fear, the conversation has become polarized. I am sorry to say:

- I hear scandals about the over-prescribing of MHT.
- I see fearmongering about potential health-risks both of MHT and of menopause itself.
- I see social media influencers mocking others who are speaking on these platforms.
- Wild promises about anything from medicines to supplements to diets are being made by private doctors and by more holistic support providers.
- Pain-points like weight-gain are being overtly used as a target to bring in business.
- Individuals on chat groups, etc., who have no qualifications are evangelically shouting about the benefits they have experienced from anything from MHT to diets or supplements, and deriding those who choose differently.
- Women without qualifications are advising others on chat groups about how much topical MHT they should use.

- There has been a *huge* surge in the number of things being sold to women in menopause.

Far from happy that we are now in a better world for menopause, or that my girls will be, I wonder will there be even more pressure not to "succumb" to this change? Will menopause be even more medicalized? Will there be more expectation that only MHT can protect health? Or will there be an even more dizzying array of concoctions claiming to fix things? Will my girls feel inferior if they don't "control" their symptoms, stay in the same body shape of their 20s and 30s, "look and feel years younger", have fab social lives and regular sex, and continue to work their asses off instead of honoring their need to rest and change?

I have fears and I have hopes.

My hopes lie in you. Thank you for reading this book, as a step toward helping women find clarity, understanding, and a sense of support, from which they may be able to find the voice they are asked to quiet in our society, to advocate for their own needs, and perhaps to make the menopausal journey an easier one for the women coming up behind.

> *i stand*
> *on the sacrifices*
> *of a million women before me*
> *thinking*
> *what can i do*
> *to make this mountain taller*
> *so the women after me*
> *can see farther*
>
> *– legacy*

—Rupi Kaur

REFERENCES

Abildgaard, J., Tingstedt, J., Zhao, Y., Hartling, H.J., Tønnes Pedersen, A., Lindegaard, B., and Dam Nielsen, S. (2020). Increased systemic inflammation and altered distribution of T-cell subsets in postmenopausal women. *PLoS One* 15(6). doi: 10.1371/journal.pone.0235174.

Angelou, K., Grigoriadis, T., Diakosavvas, M., Zacharakis, D., and Athanasiou, S. (2020). The Genitourinary Syndrome of Menopause: An Overview of the Recent Data, *Cureus* 12(4). doi: 10.7759/cureus.7586.

Appleton, B. (1996). *Stretching and Flexibility: Everything You Never Wanted to Know*. Available at: https://web.mit.edu/tkd/stretch/stretching_toc.html

Bacon, L., and Aphramor, L. (2011). Weight Science: Evaluating the Evidence for a Paradigm Shift. Challenging assumptions in obesity research, *Nutrition Journal* 10(9). doi.org/10.1186/1475-2891-10-9

Bernardes, B.T., Magalhães Resende, A.P., Stüpp, L., Oliveira, E., Castro, R.A., Jármy di Bella, Z.I.K., M.J.B., and Ferreira Sartori, M.G. (2012). Efficacy of pelvic floor muscle training and hypopressive exercises for treating pelvic organ prolapse in women: randomized controlled trial, *Sao Paulo Medical Journal* 130(1): 5-9. doi: 10.1590/s1516-31802012000100002

Bridges, L., and Sharma, M. (2017). The Efficacy of Yoga as a Form of Treatment for Depression, *Journal of Evidence-Based Complementary and Alternative Medicine* 22(4): 1017–1028. doi: 10.1177/2156587217715927

British Menopause Society (2022). Joint position statement by the British Menopause Society, Royal College of Obstetricians and Gynaecologists and Society for Endocrinology on best practice recommendations for the care of women experiencing the menopause. *Post Reproductive Health* 28(3): 123–125. doi: 10.1177/20533691221104879.

Budhi, R.B., Payghan, S., and Deepeshwar, S. (2019). Changes in Lung Function Measures Following Bhastrika Pranayama (Bellows Breath) and Running in Healthy Individuals, *International Journal of Yoga* 12(3): 233-239. doi: 10.4103/ijoy.IJOY_43_18

Cabanas-Sánchez, V., Esteban-Cornejo, I., Parra-Soto, S., Petermann-Rocha, F., Gray, S.R., Rodríguez-Artalejo, F., Ho, F.K.,

Pell, J.P., Martínez-Gómez, D., and Celis-Morales, C. (2022). Muscle strength and incidence of depression and anxiety: findings from the UK Biobank prospective cohort study, *Journal of Cachexia, Sarcopenia and Muscle* 13(4): 1983-94. doi: 10.1002/jcsm.12963

Calman, B., and Adams, S. (2023). Leading menopause doctor is accused of risking women's health with 'alarmingly high' doses of hormone replacement therapy. *Daily Mail* 1 April 2023.

Calton, J.B. (2010). Prevalence of micronutrient deficiency in popular diet plans. *Journal of the International Society of Sports Nutrition* 7(24). doi: 10.1186/1550-2783-7-24

Chen, J., Geng, L., Song, X., Li, H., Giordan, N., and Liao, O. (2013). Evaluation of the efficacy and safety of hyaluronic acid vaginal gel to ease vaginal dryness: a multicenter, randomized, controlled, open-label, parallel-group, clinical trial. *The Journal of Sexual Medicine* 10(6): 1575-84. doi: 10.1111/jsm.12125.

Chen, M.N., Lin, C.C., and Liu, C.F. (2020). Efficacy of phytoestrogens for menopausal symptoms: a meta-analysis and systematic review, *Climacteric* 18(2): 260-69. doi: 10.3109/13697137.2014.966241

Clark, K.L., Klaus, W., Flechsenhar, R., Aukermann, D.F., Meza, F., Millard, R.L., Deitch, J.R., Sherbondy, P.S., and Albert, A. (2008). 24-Week study on the use of collagen hydrolysate as a dietary supplement in athletes with activity-related joint pain, *Current Medical Research and Opinion* 24(5): 1485-96. doi: 10.1185/030079908x291967

Colombarolli, M.S., de Oliveira, J., and Cordás, T.A. (2022). Craving for carbs: food craving and disordered eating in low-carb dieters and its association with intermittent fasting. *Eating and Weight Disorders* 27(8): 3109–17. https://doi.org/10.1007/s40519-022-01437-z

Cortes, Y.I., Coslov, N., Richardson, M.K., and Woods, N.F. (2023). Symptom experience during the late reproductive stage versus the menopausal transition in the Spanish-language Women Living Better survey, *Menopause* 30(3): 260-66. doi: 10.1097/GME.0000000000002132

Coslov, N., Richardson, M.K., and Woods, N.F. (2021). Symptom experience during the late reproductive stage and the menopausal transition: observations from the Women Living Better survey, *Menopause* 28(9): 1012-25. doi: 10.1097/GME.0000000000001805

Coyle, D. (2018). Intermittent Fasting For Women: A Beginner's Guide, *Healthline* July 22. Retrieved from https://www.healthline.com/nutrition/intermittent-fasting-for-women, 09.05.23.

Craft, B.B., Carroll, H.A., and Lustyk, M.K. (2016). Gender differences in exercise habits and quality of life reports: assessing the moderating effects of reasons for exercise, *International Journal of Liberal Arts and Social Science* 2(5): 65-76. PMID: 27668243

Cramer, H., Peng, W., and Lauche, R. (2018). Yoga for menopausal symptoms— A systematic review and meta-analysis, *Maturitas* 109: 13-25. doi: 10.1016/j.maturitas.2017.12.005

Della Torre, S., Rando, G., Meda, C., Stell, A., Chambon, P., Krust, A., Ibarra, C., Magni, P., Ciana, P., and Maggi, A. (2011). Amino acid-dependent activation of liver estrogen receptor alpha integrates metabolic and reproductive functions via IGF-1, *Cell Metabolism* 13(2): 205-14. doi: 10.1016/j.cmet.2011.01.002

Dharmayani, P.N.A., Juergens, M., Allman-Farinelli, M., and Mihrshahi, S. (2021). Association between fruit and vegetable consumption and depression symptoms in young people and adults aged 15–45: A systematic review of cohort studies, *International Journal of Environmental Research and Public Health* 18(2): 780. doi: 10.3390/ijerph18020780

Dhikav, V., Karmarkar, G., Gupta, R., Verma, M., Gupta, R., Gupta, S., and Anand, K.S. (2010). Yoga in female sexual functions, *Journal of Sexual Medicine* 7(2.2): 964-70. doi: 10.1111/j.1743-6109.2009.01580.x

Djalilova, D.M., Schulz, P.S., Berger, A.M., Case, A.J., Kupzyk, K.A., Ross, A.C. (2018). Impact of yoga on inflammatory biomarkers: A systematic review, *Biological Research for Nursing* 21(2): 198-209. doi:10.1177/1099800418820162

Enns, D.L., and Tiidus, P.M. (2010). The influence of estrogen on skeletal muscle, *Sports Medicine* 40: 41–58. https://doi.org/10.2165/11319760-000000000-00000

Eyre, H.A., Siddarth, P., Van Dyk, B.A.K., Paholpak, P., Ercoli, L., St Cyr, N., Yang, H., Khalsa, D.S., and Lavretsky, H. (2017). A randomized controlled trial of Kundalini yoga in mild cognitive impairment, *International Psychogeriatrics* 29(4): 557-67. doi: 10.1017/S1041610216002155

Falkenberg, R.I., Eising, C., and Peters, M.L. (2018). Yoga and immune system functioning: a systematic review of randomized controlled trials, *Journal of Behavioural Medicine* 41(4): 467-82. doi: 10.1007/s10865-018-9914-y

Fede, C., Pirri, C., Fan, C., Albertin, G., Porzionato, A., Macchi, V., De Caro, R., and Stecco, C. (2019). Sensitivity of the fasciae to sex hormone levels: Modulation of collagen-I, collagen-III and fibrillin production, *PLoS One* 14(9): e0223195. doi: 10.1371/journal.pone.0223195

Fensham, N.C., Heikura, I.A., McKay, A.K.A., Tee, N., Ackerman, K.E., and Burke, L.M. (2022). Short-term carbohydrate restriction impairs bone formation at rest and during prolonged exercise to a greater degree than low energy availability, *Journal of Bone and Mineral Research* 37(10): 1915-25. doi: 10.1002/jbmr.4658

Fernández-Rodríguez, R., Alvarez-Bueno, C., Reina-Gutiérrez, S., Torres-Costoso, A., de Arenas-Arroyo, S.N., and Martínez-Vizcaíno, V. (2021). Effectiveness of Pilates and Yoga to improve bone density in adult women: A systematic review and meta-analysis, *PLoS One* 16(5): e0251391. doi: 10.1371/journal.pone.0251391

Ferreira-Vorkapic, C., Borba-Pinheiro, C.J., Marchioro, M., and Santana, D. (2018). The impact of Yoga Nidra and seated on the mental health of college professors, *International Journal of Yoga* 11(3): 215–23. doi: 10.4103/ijoy.IJOY_57_17

Flaherty, M. (2020). *Does Yoga Work? Answers from Science.* Independently published: Amazon.

Fugate Woods, N., Sullivan Mitchell, E., and Smith-DiJulio, K. (2009). Cortisol levels during the menopausal transition and early postmenopause: observations from the Seattle Midlife Women's Health Study, *Menopause* 16(4): 708-18. doi: 10.1097/gme.0b013e318198d6b2

García-Coronado, J.M., Martínez-Olvera, L., Elizondo-Omaña, R.E., Acosta-Olivo, C.A., Vilchez-Cavazos, F., Simental-Mendía, L.E., and Simental-Mendía, M. (2019). Effect of collagen supplementation on osteoarthritis symptoms: a meta-analysis of randomized placebo-controlled trials, *International Orthopaedics* 43(3): 531-38. doi: 10.1007/s00264-018-4211-5

Garmy-Susini, B. (2019). Hormone therapy outcome in lymphedema, *Aging* 11(2): 291–92. doi: 10.18632/aging.101772

Gibson, C.J., Huang, A.J., McCaw, B., Subak, L.L., Thom, D.H., and Van Den Eeden, S.K. (2019). Associations of intimate partner violence, sexual assault, and posttraumatic stress disorder with menopause symptoms among midlife and older women. *JAMA Internal Medicine* 179(1): 80-87. doi:10.1001/jamainternmed.2018.5233

Grave, R.D. (2020). Regular eating, not intermittent fasting, is the best strategy for a healthy eating control. *Italian Journal of Eating Disorders and Obesity* 2: 5-7. doi: 10.32044/ijedo.2020.02

Harte, J.L., Eifert, G.H., and Smith, R. (1995). The effects of running and meditation on beta-endorphin, corticotropin-releasing hormone and cortisol in plasma, and on mood, *Biological Psychology* 40(3): 251-65. doi: 10.1016/0301-0511(95)05118-t

Harvard Health (2021). Osteopenia: When you have weak bones, but not osteoporosis. Harvard Health Publishing. Retrieved from https://www.health.harvard.edu/womens-health/osteopenia-when-you-have-weak-bones-but-not-osteoporosis, 09.09.23

Heeter, C., Allbritton, M., Lehto, R., Miller, P., McDaniel, P., and Paletta, M. (2021). Feasibility, acceptability, and outcomes of a yoga-based meditation intervention for hospice professionals to combat burnout, *International Journal of Environmental Research and Public Health* 18(5): 2515. doi: 10.3390/ijerph18052515

Heikura, I.A., Burke, L.M., Hawley, J.A., Ross, M.L., Garvican Lewis, L., Sharma, A.P., McKay, A.K.A., Leckey, J.J., Welvaert, M., McCall, L., and Ackerman, K.E. (2020). A short-term ketogenic diet impairs markers of bone health in response to exercise, *Frontiers in Endocrinology* 10: 880. https://doi.org/10.3389/fendo.2019.00880

Hong, A.R., and Kim, S.W. (2018). Effects of resistance exercise on bone health, *Endocrinology and Metabolism* 33(4): 435–444. doi: 10.3803/EnM.2018.33.4.435

Huang, A.J., Phillips, S., Schembri, M., Vittinghoff, E., and Grady, D. (2015). Device-guided slow-paced respiration for menopausal hot flushes: A Randomized controlled trial, *Obstetrics and Gynaecology* 125(5): 1130-1138. doi: 10.1097/AOG.0000000000000821.

Hunter, M., and Smith, M. (2017). Cognitive Behaviour Therapy (CBT) for menopausal symptoms. Information for women (in collaboration with the British Menopause Society). *Post Reproductive Health* 23(2): 77-82. doi:10.1177/2053369117711635

Iacono, D., Markesbery, W.R., Gross, M., Pletnikova, O., Rudow, G., Zandi. P., and Troncoso, J.C. (2009). The Nun study: clinically silent AD, neuronal hypertrophy, and linguistic skills in early life. *Neurology* 73(9): 665-73.

Innes, K.E., Selfe, T.K., Brundage, K., Montgomery, C., Wen, S., Kandati, S., Bowles, H., Khalsa, D.S., and Huysmans, Z. (2018). Effects of meditation and music-listening on blood biomarkers of cellular aging and Alzheimer's disease in adults with subjective cognitive decline: an exploratory randomized clinical trial, *Journal of Alzheimer's Dementia* 66(3): 947-970. doi: 10.3233/JAD-180164

Kadachha, D., Soni, N., and Parekh, A. (2016). Effects of yogasana on balance in geriatric population, *International Journal of Physiotherapy and Research* 4(2): 1401-07. http://dx.doi.org/10.16965/ijpr.2016.107

Kaji, H. (2014). Interaction between muscle and bone, *Journal of Bone Metabolism* 21(1): 29–40. doi: 10.11005/jbm.2014.21.1.29

Kapoor, E., Okuno, M., Miller, V.M., Rocca, L.G., Rocca, W.A., Kling, J.M., Kuhle, C.L., Mara, K.C., Enders, F.T., and Faubion, S.S. (2020). Association of adverse childhood experiences with menopausal symptoms: results from the data registry on experiences of aging, Menopause and Sexuality (DREAMS), *Maturitas* 143: 209-15. doi: 10.1016/j.maturitas.2020.10.006

Kaur, N., Majumdar, V., Nagarathna, R., Malik, N., Anand, A., and Nagendra, H.R. (2021). Diabetic yoga protocol improves glycemic, anthropometric and lipid levels in high risk individuals for diabetes: a randomized controlled trial from Northern India, *Diabetology & Metabolic Syndrome* 13, 149. https://doi.org/10.1186/s13098-021-00761-1

Khalsa, D.S., and Newberg, A.B. (2021). Spiritual fitness: a new dimension in Alzheimer's Disease prevention, *Journal of Alzheimer's Disease* 80(2): 505-19. doi: 10.3233/JAD-201433

Kjaer, T.W., Bertelsen, C., Piccini, P., Brooks, D., Alving, J., and Lou, H.C. (2002). Increased dopamine tone during meditation-induced change of consciousness, *Cognitive Brain*

Research 13(2): 255-59. doi: 10.1016/s0926-6410(01)00106-9.

Krishna, B.H., Keerthi, G.S., Kumar, C.K., and Reddy, N.M. (2015). Association of leukocyte telomere length with oxidative stress in yoga practitioners, *Journal of Clinical Diagnostic Research* 9(3): CC01–CC03. doi: 10.7860/JCDR/2015/13076.5729

Leblanc, D.R., Schneider, M., Angele, P., Vollmer, G., and Docheva, D. (2017). The effect of estrogen on tendon and ligament metabolism and function, *The Journal of Steroid Biochemistry and Molecular Biology* 172:106-16. https://doi.org/10.1016/j.jsbmb.2017.06.008

Lee, M.S., Kim, J.I., Ha, J.Y., Boddy, K., Ernst, E. (2009). Yoga for menopausal symptoms: a systematic review *Menopause Journal* 16(3): 602-08. doi: 10.1097/gme.0b013e31818ffe39

Lee, M., Huntoon, E.A., and Sinaki, M. (2019). Soft tissue and bony injuries attributed to the practice of yoga: a biomechanical analysis and implications for management, *Mayo Clinic* 94(3): 424-31. https://doi.org/10.1016/j.mayocp.2018.09.024

Leow, Z.Z., Guelfi, K.J., Davis, E.A., Jones, T.W., and Fournier, P.A. (2018). The glycaemic benefits of a very-low-carbohydrate ketogenic diet in adults with Type 1 diabetes mellitus may be opposed by increased hypoglycaemia risk and dyslipidaemia, *Diabetic Medicine: Journal of British Diabetic Association*. doi: 10.1111/dme.13663

Lin, S.L., Huang, C.Y., Shiu, S.P., and Yeh, S.H. (2015). Effects of yoga on stress, stress adaption, and heart rate variability among mental health professionals—a randomized controlled trial, *Worldviews on Evidence-Based Nursing* 12(4): 236–45. doi/pdf/10.1111/wvn.12097

Lopes, J.S.S., Machado, A.F., Micheletti, J.K., de Almeida, A.C., Cavina, A.P., and Pastre, C.M. (2019). Effects of training with elastic resistance versus conventional resistance on muscular strength: A systematic review and meta-analysis, *Sage Open Medicine* 7. doi: 10.1177/2050312119831116

Lu, L.Y.H., Rosner, B., Chang, G., and Fishman, L.M. (2015). Twelve-minute daily yoga regimen reverses osteoporotic bone loss, *Topics in Geriatric Rehabilitation* 32(2): 81-87. doi: 10.1097/TGR.0000000000000085

Lu, X., Liu, L., and Yuan, R. (2020). Effect of the information support method combined with yoga exercise on the depression, anxiety, and sleep quality of menopausal women, *Psychiatria Danubina* 32(3-4): 380-88. doi: 10.24869/psyd.2020.380

Madanmohan, Thombre, D.P., Balakumar, B., Nambinarayanan, T.K., Thakur, S., Krishnamurthy, N., and Chandrabose, A. (1992). Effect of yoga training on reaction time, respiratory endurance and muscle strength, *Indian Journal of Physiology and Pharmacology* 36(4): 229-33.

Malhotra, V., Javed, D., Wakode, S., Bharshankar, R., Soni, N., and Porter, P.K.

(2022). Study of immediate neurological and autonomic changes during kapalbhati pranayama in yoga practitioners, *Journal of Family Medicine and Primary Care* 11(2): 720-27. doi: 10.4103/jfmpc.jfmpc_1662_21

Malutan, A.M., Dan, M., Nicolae, C., and Carmen, M. (2014). Proinflammatory and anti-inflammatory cytokine changes related to menopause, *Menopause review* 13(3): 162–168. doi: 10.5114/pm.2014.43818

Mann, E., Smith, M.J., Hellier, J., Balabanovic, J.A., Hamed, H., Grunfeld, E.A., and Hunter, M.S. (2012). Cognitive behavioural treatment for women who have menopausal symptoms after breast cancer treatment (MENOS 1): a randomised controlled trial, *Lancet Oncology* 3(3): 309-18. doi: 10.1016/S1470-2045(11)70364-3

Marques, A., Gomez-Baya, D., Peralta, M., Frasquilho, D., Santos, T., Martins, J., Ferrari, G., and Gaspar de Matos, M. (2020), The effect of muscular strength on depression symptoms in adults: a systematic review and meta-analysis, *International Journal of Environmental Research and Public Health* 17(16): 5674. doi: 10.3390/ijerph17165674

Mayo Clinic (2021). Chronic stress puts your health at risk. https://www.mayoclinic.org/healthy-lifestyle/stress-management/in-depth/stress/art-20046037. Accessed 09.06.23.

Menopause Society, The (2022). The 2022 hormone therapy position statement of The North American Menopause Society. *Menopause: The Journal of The North American Menopause Society* 29(7): 767-94. doi: 10.1097/GME.0000000000002028

Minkin, M.J., Reiter, S., and Maamari, R. (2015). Prevalence of postmenopausal symptoms in North America and Europe, *Menopause* 22(11): 1231-38. doi: 10.1097/GME.0000000000000464

Mizuhashi, F., and Koide, K. (2020). Salivary secretion and salivary stress hormone level changes induced by tongue rotation exercise, *Journal of Advance Prosthodontics* 12(4): 204-09. doi: 10.4047/jap.2020.12.4.204

Mosconi, L., Berti, V., Dyke, J., Schelbaum, E., Jett, S., Loughlin, L., Jang, G., Rahman, A., Hristov, H., Pahlajani, S., Andrews, R., Matthews, D., Etingin, O., Ganzer, C., de Leon, M., Isaacson, R., and Diaz Brinton, R. (2021). Menopause impacts human brain structure, connectivity, energy metabolism, and amyloid-beta deposition, *Scientific Reports* 11, 10867. https://doi.org/10.1038/s41598-021-90084-y

Navarro-Brazález, B. Prieto-Gómez, V., Prieto-Merino, D., Sánchez-Sánchez, B., McLean, L., and Torres-Lacomba, M. (2020). Effectiveness of Hypopressive exercises in women with pelvic floor dysfunction: a randomised controlled trial, *Journal of Clinical Medicine* 9(4): 1149. doi: 10.3390/jcm9041149

Negrete-Corona, J., Alvarado-Soriano, J.C., and Reyes-Santiago, L.A. (2014). Hip fracture as risk factor for mortality in patients over 65 years of age. Case-control study, *Acta Ortopedico Mexicana* 28(6): 352-62.

Neratinni, M., Jett, S., Andy, C., Carlton. C., Zarate. C., Boneu. C., Battista. M., Pahlajani, S., Loeb-Zeitlin, S., Havryulik, Y., Williams, S., Christos, P., Fink, M., Diaz Brinton, R., Mosconi, L. (2023). Systematic review and meta-analysis of the effects of menopause hormone therapy on risk of Alzheimer's disease and dementia, *Frontiers in Aging Neuroscience* 15. doi: 10.3389/fnagi.2023.1260427

Newton, K.M., Reed, S.D., Guthrie, K.A., Sherman, K.J, Booth-LaForce, C., Caan, B., Sternfeld, B., Carpenter, J.S., Learman, L.A., Freeman, E.W., Cohen, L.S., Joffe, H., Anderson, G.L., Larson, J.C., Hunt, J.R., Ensrud, K.E., and LaCroix, A.Z. (2015). Efficacy of yoga for vasomotor symptoms: a randomized controlled trial, *Menopause* 21(4): 339-46. doi: 10.1097/GME.0b013e31829e4baa

Norton, S., Chilcot, J., and Hunter, M. (2014). Cognitive-behavior therapy for menopausal symptoms (hot flushes and night sweats): moderators and mediators of treatment effects, *Menopause* 21(6): 574-78. doi:10.1097/GME.0000000000000095

Parkin, A., Parker, A., and Dagnall, N. (2017). Effects of handedness & saccadic bilateral eye movements on the specificity of past autobiographical memory & episodic future thinking, *Brain and Cognition* 114: 40-51. doi: 10.1016/j.bandc.2017.03.006

Parker, A., Parkin, A., and Dagnall, N. (2023). Effects of saccadic eye movements on episodic & semantic memory fluency in older and younger participants, *Memory* 31(1): 34-46. doi: 10.1080/09658211.2022.2122997

Parkinson, C. (2019). Yoga teachers 'risking serious hip problems', BBC News website, Nov 3, 2019. Available at www.bbc.com/news/health-50181155. Accessed 09.06.23.

Patil, D.C., and Honkalas, P. (2022). The impact of kapalabhati on menopausal women's pelvic floor muscle strength, *Journal of Community Health Management* 9(4): 178-82.

Perry, S. (2019). Ehlers-Danlos Syndrome and hEDS symptoms in menopause, Gennev, Dec 10, 2019. Available at www.gennev.com/education/heds-symptoms. Accessed 09.06.23.

Prior, J.C. (1998). Perimenopause: the complex endocrinology of the menopausal transition, *Endocrine Reviews* 19(4): 397-428. https://doi.org/10.1210/edrv.19.4.0341

Rapaport, L. (2015). Culture may influence how women experience menopause, Reuters, June 5, 2015. Available at www.reuters.com/article/us-health-menopause-perceptions-idUSKBN0OL1XH20150605. Accessed 09.06.23.

Rinonapoli, G.. Ruggiero, C., Meccariello, L., Bisaccia, M., Ceccarini, P., and Caraffa, A. (2021). Osteoporosis in men: a review of an underestimated bone condition, *International Journal of Molecular Science* 22(4): 2105. doi: 10.3390/ijms22042105

Robert, B. (2008). Roughly one quarter of U.S. women affected by pelvic floor disorders, National Institutes of Health, Sept 17, 2008. Available at www.nih.gov/news-events/news-releases/roughly-one-quarter-us-women-affected-pelvic-floor-disorders. Accessed 09.06.23.

Roman-Blass, J.A., Castañeda, S., Largo, R., and Herrero-Beaumont, G. (2009). Osteoarthritis associated with estrogen deficiency, *Arthritis Research and Therapy* 11(5): 241. doi: 10.1186/ar2791

Santoro, N. (1996). Characterization of reproductive hormonal dynamics in the perimenopause. *Journal of Clinical Endocrinology and Metabolism* 81(4): 1495-501. doi: 10.1210/jcem.81.4.8636357.

Saoji, A.A., Raghavendra, B.R., and Manjunath, N.K. (2019). Effects of yogic breath regulation: A narrative review of scientific evidence, *Journal of Ayurveda and Integrative Medicine* 10(1): 50-58. https://doi.org/10.1016/j.jaim.2017.07.008

Sauer, T., Sykes Tottenham, L., Ethier, A., and Gordon, J.L. (2020). Perimenopausal vasomotor symptoms and the cortisol awakening response, *Menopause* 27(11): 1322-27. doi: 10.1097/GME.0000000000001588

Sfeir, J.G., Drake, M.T., Sonawane, V.J., and Sinaki, M. (2018). Vertebral compression fractures associated with yoga: a case series, *European Journal of Physical and Rehabilitation Medicine* 54(6): 947-51. doi: 10.23736/S1973-9087.18.05034-7

Shobana, R., Maheshkumar, K., Venkateswaran, S.T., Bagavad Geetha, M., and Padmavathi, R. (2022). Effect of long-term yoga training on autonomic function among the healthy adults, *Journal of Family Medicine and Primary Care* 11(7): 3471-75. doi: 10.4103/jfmpc.jfmpc_199_21

Shohani, M., Badfar, G., Nasirkandy, M.P., Kaikhavani, S., Rahmati, S., Modmeli, Y., Soleymani, A., and Azami, M. (2018). The effect of yoga on stress, anxiety, and depression in women, *International Journal of Preventative Medicine* 9(1): 21. doi: 10.4103/ijpvm.IJPVM_242_16

Simm, P.J., Bicknell-Royle, J., Lawrie, J., Nation, J., Draffin, K., Stewart, K.G., Cameron, F.J., Scheffer, I.E., and Mackay, M.T. (2017). The effect of the ketogenic diet on the developing skeleton, *Epilepsy Research* 136: 62-66. doi: 10.1016/j.eplepsyres.2017.07.014

Sinaki, M., Itoi, E., Wahner, H.W., Wollan, P., Gelzcer, R., Mullan, B.P., Collins, D.A., and Hodgson, S.F. (2002). Stronger back muscles reduce the incidence of vertebral fractures: a prospective 10 year follow-up of postmenopausal women, *Bone* 30(6): 836-41. doi: 10.1016/s8756-3282(02)00739-1

Smith, L. (2022). 41 yoga statistics: how many people practice yoga? The Good Body. Available at www.thegoodbody.com/yoga-statistics. Acessed 06.09.23.

Smith, L.L., Brunetz, M.H., Chenier, T.C., McCammon, M.R., Houmard, J.A., Franklin, M.E., and Israel, R.G. (1993). The effects of static and ballistic stretching on delayed onset muscle soreness and creatine kinase, *Research Quarterly* for Exercise and Sport 64(1): 103-107. doi: 10.1080/02701367.1993.10608784

Söderkvist, S., Ohlén, K., and Dimberg, U. (2017). How the experience of emotion is modulated by facial feedback, *Journal of Nonverbal Behaviour* 42(1): 129-51. doi: 10.1007/s10919-017-0264-1

Sood, R., Sood, A., Wolf, S.L., Linquist, B.M., Liu, H., Sloan, J.A., Satele, D.V., Loprinzi, C.L., and Barton, D.L. (2013). Paced breathing compared with usual breathing for hot flashes, *Menopause* 20(2) :179-84. doi: 10.1097/gme.0b013e31826934b6

Souza, L.A., Reis, I.A., and Lima, A.A. (2022). Climacteric symptoms and quality of life in yoga practitioners, *Explore* 18(1): 70-75. doi: 10.1016/j.explore.2020.09.005

Späth-Schwalbe, E., Schöller, T., Kern, W., Fehm, H.L., and Born, J., (1992). Nocturnal adrenocorticotropin and cortisol secretion depends on sleep duration and decreases in association with spontaneous awakening in the morning, *Journal of Clinical Endocrinology and Metabolism* 75(6): 1431-35. doi: 10.1210/jcem.75.6.1334495.

Stine, J.G., DiJoseph, K., Pattison, Z., Harrington, A., Chinchilli, V.M. Schmitz, K. H., and Loomba, R. (2023). Exercise training is associated with treatment response in liver fat content by magnetic resonance imaging independent of clinically significant body weight loss in patients with nonalcoholic fatty liver disease: a systematic review and meta-analysis, *American Journal of Gastroenterology* 118(7): 1204-13. doi: 10.14309/ajg.0000000000002098

Streeter, C.C., Whitfield, T.H., Owen, L., Rein, T., Karri, S.K., Yakhkind, A., Perlmutter, R., Prescot, A., Renshaw, P.F., Ciraulo, D.A., and Jensen, J.E. (2010). Effects of yoga versus walking on mood, anxiety, and brain GABA levels: a randomized controlled MRS study, *Journal of Alternative and Complimentary Medicine* 16(11): 1145–52. doi: 10.1089/acm.2010.0007

Streeter, C.C., Gerbarg, P.L., Whitfield, T.H., Owen, L., Johnston, J., Silveri, M.M., Gensler, M., Faulkner, C.L., Mann, C., Wixted, M., Hernon, A.M., Nyer, M.B., Brown, E.R., Jensen, J.E. (2017). Treatment of major depressive disorder with Iyengar yoga and coherent breathing: a randomized controlled dosing study, *Journal of Alternative and Complimentary Medicine* 23(3): 201-07. doi: 10.1089/acm.2016.0140

Sturgiss, E., Jay, M., Campbell-Scherer, D., and van Weel, C. (2017). Challenging assumptions in obesity research, *BMJ* 359: j5303. doi: 10.1136/bmj.j5303

Swain, T.A., and McGwin, G. (2016). Yoga-related injuries in the United States from 2001 to 2014. Orthopaedic Journal of Sports Medicine 4(11): 2325967116671703. doi: 10.1177/2325967116671703

Thirthalli, J., Naveen, G.H., Rao, M.G., Varambally, S., Christopher, R., and Gangadhar, B.N. (2013). Cortisol and antidepressant effects of yoga, *Indian Journal of Psychiatry* 55(Suppl 3): S405-S408. doi: 10.4103/0019-5545.116315

Thomas, B. (2016). A new paradigm of anatomy with John Sharkey, *Liberated Being* podcast, ep. 55. https://podcasts.apple.com/us/podcast/ep-55-a-new-paradigm-of-anatomy-with-john-sharkey/id885440301?i=1000368858312

Tiidus, P.M., (2003). Influence of estrogen on skeletal muscle damage, inflammation, and repair, *Exercise and Sport Sciences Reviews* 31(1): 40-44. doi: 10.1097/00003677-200301000-00008

Tolahunase, M., Sagar, R., and Dada, R. (2017). Impact of yoga and meditation on cellular aging in apparently healthy individuals: a prospective, open-label single-arm exploratory study, *Oxidative Medicine and Cellular Longevity* 2017: 7928981. doi: 10.1155/2017/7928981

Tomasevic-Todorovic, S., Vazic, A., Issaka, A., and Hanna, F. (2018). Comparative assessment of fracture risk among osteoporosis and osteopenia patients: a cross-sectional study, *Open Access Rheumatology* 10: 61–66. doi: 10.2147/OARRR.S151307

Tooley, G.A., Armstrong, S.M., Norman, T.R., and Sali, A. (2000). Acute increases in night-time plasma melatonin levels following a period of meditation, *Biological Psychology* 53(1): 69-78. doi.org/10.1016/S0301-0511(00)00035-1

Toprak, N., Sen, S., and Varhan, B. (2021). The role of diaphragmatic breathing exercise on urinary incontinence treatment: A pilot study, *Journal of Bodywork and Movement Therapies* 29: 146-153. doi: 10.1016/j.jbmt.2021.10.002.

Triebner, K., Matulonga, B., Johannessen, A., Suske, S., Benediktsdóttir, B., Demoly P., Dharmage, S.C., Franklin, K.A., Garcia-Aymerich, J., Blanco, J.A.G., and Heinrich, J. (2016). Menopause is associated with accelerated lung function decline, *American Journal of Respiratory and Critical Care Medicine* 195(8): 1058-65. doi: 10.1164/rccm.201605-0968OC

Uvnas-Moberg, K., and Petersson, M. (2005). Oxytocin, a mediator of anti-stress, well-being, social interaction, growth and healing, *Zeitschrift fur Psychosomatische Medizin und Psychotherapie* 51(1): 57-80. doi: 10.13109/zptm.2005.51.1.57

van Aalst, J., Ceccarini, J., Demyttenaere, K., Sunaert, S. and Van Laere, K. (2020). What has neuroimaging taught us on the neurobiology of yoga? A review. *Frontiers in Integrative Neuroscience* 14: 34. doi: 10.3389/fnint.2020.00034

Wang, W.L., Chen, K.H., and Pan, Y.C. (2020). The effect of yoga on sleep quality and insomnia in women with sleep problems: a systematic review and meta-analysis. *BMC Psychiatry* 20, 195. https://doi.org/10.1186/s12888-020-02566-4

Watson, S.L., Weeks, B.K., Weis, L.J., Harding, A.T. Horan, S.A., and Beck, B.R. (2017). High-intensity resistance and impact training improves bone mineral density and physical function in postmenopausal women with osteopenia and osteoporosis: the LIFTMOR randomized controlled trial, *American Society for Bone and Mineral Research* 33(2): 211-20. https://doi.org/10.1002/jbmr.3284

White, A., and Cherney, K. (2021). Are phytoestrogens good for you? Healthline, June 2021. Available at www.healthline.com/health/phytoestrogens. Accessed 09.06.23.

WHO (2022). Menopause. Available at www.who.int/news-room/fact-sheets/detail/menopause. Accessed 09.06.23.

Wibisono, C., Rowe, N., Beavis, E., Kepreotes, H., Mackie, F.E., Lawson, J.A., and Cardamone, M. (2015). Ten-year single-center experience of the ketogenic diet: factors influencing efficacy, tolerability, and compliance, *The Journal of Paediatrics* 166(4): 1030-6.e1. doi: 10.1016/j.jpeds.2014.12.018

Wluka, A.E., Wolfe, R., Davis, S.R., Stuckey, S., and Cicuttini, F.M. (2003). Tibial cartilage volume change in healthy postmenopausal women: a longitudinal study, *Annals of the Rheumatic Diseases* 63: 444-49. http://dx.doi.org/10.1136/ard.2003.008433

Wyon, M.A., Smith, A., and Koutedakis, Y. (2013). A comparison of strength and stretch interventions on active and passive ranges of movement in dancers: a randomised controlled trial, *Journal of Strength and Conditioning Research* 27(11): 3053-59.

Zaied, N.F.F., Taman, A.H.S., Hassan, T., Alam, M., and Roma, N.Z.H. (2021). Effect of paced breathing technique on hot flashes and quality of daily life activities among surgically menopaused women, *Egyptian Journal of Health Care* 10(4): 693-706. doi: 10.21608/ejhc.2019.266502

Zhao, R., Zhao, M., and Xu, Z. (2015). The effects of differing resistance training modes on the preservation of bone mineral density in postmenopausal women: a meta-analysis, *Osteoporosis International* 26(5): 1605-18. doi: 10.1007/s00198-015-3034-0

INDEX

abdominal massage, 178–179
aching joints, 171–172
acopia, 168
allostatic load, 28
Alzheimer's disease, 26, 128–129. *See also* brain
angel twists, 58–59. *See also* somatic movement
antioxidants, 186
anxiety, 159
    addressing, 160
    CBT for, 162
    mind-body techniques for managing, 162–163
    tools for easing, 161
arm float, 56. *See also* somatic movement
asana practice, change in, 70. *See also* yoga class structure
    body areas vulnerable to injury, 71
    exercise in general, 72–73
    functional yoga, 73–74
    inflammation and joint health, 71
    reasons for considering, 70
    reimagining yoga postures, 73–74
    stretching, 74–88
asanas/poses
    adding muscular challenge, 86
    from all-fours, 68
    angel twist, 58–59
    arm float, 56
    balancing poses, 83
    banana pose, 63
    cat/cow, 113
    child's pose, 92, 113
    cobbler, 149
    crescent lunge, 81
    dancer's pose, 84
    downward dog, 125
    downward–facing dog, 114
    eye exercises, 139–140
    half moon, 85
    half-wheel, 115
    holding a block, 148
    inversion options, 94
    locust pose, 125
    option for those who can squat, 117
    outside-in, 166–167
    pelvic tuck, 148
    pigeon pose, 82
    raised leg block hold, 149
    reclining cobbler, 90–91
    relaxing pelvic floor, 150
    safer twisting, 114
    shavasana, 97–98
    shifting mood, 165–166
    side-angle pose, 87
    side-stretch pose, 88
    sloth, or upside-down leopard on branch, 62
    slow twist, 57
    supine, 116
    for the core, 126
    triangle, 77–78, 114
    twisted deer, 95
    vestibular system challenges, 137–138
    warrior I, 124
    warrior II and III, 79–80
    yawn-stretch, 67
    yes/no, 60–61

balancing poses, 83. *See also* stretching
banana pose, 63. *See also* somatic movement
bi-lateral oophorectomy, 17
bitter foods, 183
blood sugar regulation, 188
    effects of unstable blood sugar, 188
    multi-faceted benefits of balanced blood sugar, 188–189
    nutrients, 189
    yoga for, 189
BMD. *See* bone mineral density
BMS. *See* British Menopause Society
body areas vulnerable to injury, 71
bone mineral density (BMD), 25, 110
bones, 109
    adjusting common postures, 112
    cat/cow, 113
    child's pose, 113
    common postures to avoid, 115
    downward-facing dog, 114
    exploring weights, 120–121
    getting to and from floor, 115
    half-wheel, 115
    jumping, 126–127
    maintaining bone health, 118
    nutritional guidelines for bone health, 127
    osteocalcin, 110
    osteocytes, 109
    osteogenesis, 109
    osteopenia, 109–110
    osteoporosis, 110
    posture and balance, 127
    resistance bands, 124–126

role of yoga in bone health, 111–112, 118
safer twisting, 114
sarcopenia, 110
stimulating bone, 118–127
supine, 116
triangle, 114
weight drills, 122–123
weights and resistance bands, 119
yoga safety measures, 112–117
boxed breath, 101. *See also* pranayama
brain, 128
Alzheimer's disease, 128–129
brain-related menopause symptoms, 133–134
brain snacks, 135
cognitive load, 135
eye exercises, 139–140
health in menopause, 134
map of, 133
neuroplasticity, 128
nutrition, 141
sequencing and stacking, 136
spiritual fitness, 129
stimulating, 132–135
vagus nerve, 130–131
vestibular system challenges, 137–138
yoga for brain health, 129–130
brain fog, 169–170
breathing from research-based perspective, 101. *See also* pranayama
breath practices, 150
boxed breath, 101
breathing from research-based perspective, 101
paced breath, 101
pranayama, 100–102
seasons breath, 102
watercolour breath, 101–102
British Menopause Society (BMS), 48

cardiovascular (CV), 183
disease, 25
cat/cow pose, 113
CBT. *See* cognitive behavioral therapy

CBT for Insomnia (CBTI), 161
CBTI. *See* CBT for Insomnia
"Change, The", 46
child's pose, 92, 113. *See also* restorative yoga
chronic stress, 28
cirrhosis, 182
cobbler, 149
cognitive behavioral therapy (CBT), 36, 38, 107–108. *See also* meditation
for sleep, hot flashes, and anxiety, 161–162
cognitive decline, 25–26
cognitive load, 135. *See also* brain
cortisol, 20
crescent lunge, 81. *See also* stretching
CV. *See* cardiovascular

dancer's pose, 84. *See also* stretching
diet, 191–192
Mediterranean, 141
digestive health, 177
abdominal massage, 178–179
absorption of nutrients, 180–181
digestive wellness, 177
gut-hormone connection, 177
motility, 180
nutrition, 180
yoga and movement for gut health, 180
dopamine, 64
downward dog, 125. *See also* resistance bands
downward-facing dog, 114

ECM. *See* extracellular matrix
emotional eating, 192
endorphins, 64
ER. *See* estrogen receptor
estrogen, 18, 25, 171
dominance, 23
estrogen receptor (ER), 17
estrone, 24
expectations meditation, 104–106. *See also* meditation
extracellular matrix (ECM), 70
eye exercises, 139–140. *See also* brain

fatigue, 168
fermented foods, 180
fiber-rich plant foods, 180
follicle-stimulating hormone (FSH), 19–20
food(s), 191
with anti-inflammatory properties, 185
bitter foods, 183
diet and dieting, 191–192
emotional eating, 192
fermented foods, 180
fiber-rich plant foods, 180
menopause hormone therapy, 194–197
nutrition for menopause condensed, 193
phytoestrogens, 192–193
role of health professionals in perimenopause symptoms, 197
simplified nutrition for wellness, 193–194
systemic inflammation, 185
free-radicals, 185–186
from all-fours, 68. *See also* instinctual movement
FSH. *See* follicle-stimulating hormone
functional yoga, 73–74

GABA, 27
genitourinary challenges in menopause, 143
genitourinary syndrome of menopause (GSM), 142
"Good form", 83
Grandmother Hypothesis, 107
GSM. *See* genitourinary syndrome of menopause
gut health. *See* digestive health

half moon, 85. *See also* stretching
half-wheel, 115
health
pillars of, 155
stereotypes, 39
heart health, 183
nutrition, 184
in postmenopause, 183
yoga for, 183–184
hip bandha, 82
hormesis, 40

hormone replacement therapy
(HRT), 23, 194
hormones, 17
    dopamine, 64
    endorphins, 64
    estrogen, 18, 23
    estrone, 24
    follicle-stimulating
        hormone, 19–20
    hormonal fluctuations, 23–24
    oxytocin, 64
    pleasure and feel-good
        hormones, 63–64
    progesterone, 19
    serotonin, 64
hormone therapy, 23
hot flashes, 158
    CBT for, 161–162
    practical supports, 158–159
HPA axis. *See* hypothalamus-
    pituitary-adrenal axis
HPO axis. *See* hypothalamic-
    pituitary-ovarian axis
HRT. *See* hormone replacement
    therapy
hypermobility syndrome, 75.
    See also stretching
hypopressive exercise/training,
    145
hypothalamic-pituitary-ovarian
    axis (HPO axis), 19, 20
hypothalamus-pituitary-adrenal
    axis (HPA axis), 27

IC. *See* isometric contraction
inflammation, 71, 171
    and joint health, 71
    systemic inflammation, 71,
        185–186
'information support method,
    the', 31
insoluble fibers, 180
instinctual movement, 66.
    See also mobility in
    perimenopause
    from all-fours, 68
    yawn-stretch, 67
insulin, 20
intense side-stretch pose, 88.
    See also stretching
inversion options, 94. *See also*
    restorative yoga
isometric contraction (IC), 76

joint
    health, 71
    pain, 171–172
jumping, 126–127

Kirtan Kriya meditation,
    129–130. *See also*
    meditation
Kundalini yoga (KY), 129
KY. *See* Kundalini yoga

labrum, 81
lateral arm raises, 123
late reproductive stage (LRS),
    17, 20–21, 43–44
libido changes, 174–176
liver, 181
    early signs of struggling
        liver, 182
    nutrition, 182–183
    protection, 183
    role in menopause, 181–182
    yoga for, 182
locust pose, 125. *See also*
    resistance bands
Low Pressure Training, 145
LRS. *See* late reproductive stage
lung function, 26
lymphatic system, 185, 186
    dysregulation and effects
        on women, 186
    movement stimulus, 188
    non-optimal lymphatic
        function, 186
    self-touch for lymphatic
        support, 187–188
    yoga for, 186–187

massage
    abdominal, 178–179
    Thai foot, 97–98
meditation, 99. *See also* breath
    practices; yoga class
    structure
    cognitive behavioral therapy,
        107–108
    expectations meditation,
        104–106
    guided meditations, 102–106
    Kirtan Kriya meditation,
        129–130
    perspective shifts, 106–107
    seated positions, 99

    self-advocacy meditation,
        103–104
    spaces meditation, 102–103
"Mediterranean" diet, 141
melatonin, 20
menopausal health, holistic
    approaches, 109
    bones, 109
    brain, 128
    pelvic floor, 142
menopause, 14, 17
    biochemistry of, 17
    cardiovascular disease, 25
    cognitive decline, 25–26
    cortisol, 20
    effects of chronic stress, 28
    estrogen, 18, 25
    follicle-stimulating
        hormone, 19–20
    health implications of, 25–26
    individualized care,
        community support,
        and holistic wellness,
        200
    insulin, 20
    late reproductive stage,
        20–21
    lung function, 26
    melatonin, 20
    osteoporosis, 25
    oxytocin, 20
    perimenopause, 21–24
    physical changes, body
        image, and practice
        adaptations, 199–200
    postmenopause, 24–25
    progesterone, 19
    role of stress, 27–29
    serotonin, 20
    stages of, 20–25
    testosterone, 20
    thyroid health, 26
    vision of empowerment
        and legacy, 202–203
    yoga, 31–41
    yoga session, 200–201
    yoga teachers for, 201–202
menopause hormone therapy
    (MHT), 23, 194–197
menopause, integrative
    approaches to, 155
    aching joints, 171–172
    anxiety, 159–160

brain fog, 169–170
emotional changes in perimenopause, 163–164
fatigue, 168
honoring feelings in yoga, 164–165
hot flashes, 158
libido changes, 174–176
mood-honoring additions, 164–165
outside-in, 166–167
overwhelm, 168–169
pillars of health, 155
rest and vitality, 170–171
shifting mood, 165–166
sleep, 156–158
symptoms addressed, 155
weight gain, 172–174
menopause-sensitive yoga, 48–50
menopause transition (MT), 17. *See* perimenopause
meridians, 96. *See also* restorative yoga
MHT. *See* menopause hormone therapy
micro-moving, 66. *See also* mobility in perimenopause
mobility in perimenopause, 55. *See also* yoga class structure
  improvisation in warm-up practice, 65
  instinctual movement, 66–68
  micro-moving, 66
  pleasure and feel-good hormones, 63–64
  self-led movement, 69
  somatic movement, 55–63
mood-honoring additions, 164–165
movement modality, 39
MT. *See* menopause transition
mula bandha, 144
muscular contraction types, 76. *See also* stretching
muscular engagement in yoga practice, 76. *See also* stretching
muscular inhibition, 74–75. *See also* stretching

NAMS. *See* North American Menopause Society
National Institute for Health and Care Excellence (NICE), 48
nervous system (NS), 160
neuroplasticity, 128. *See also* brain
NICE. *See* National Institute for Health and Care Excellence
non-alcoholic fatty liver disease (NAFLD), 182
non-optimal lymphatic function, 186
North American Menopause Society (NAMS), 48
NS. *See* nervous system
nutrition, 191
  for blood sugar regulation, 189
  for bone health, 127
  brain, 141
  diet and dieting, 191–192
  digestive health, 180
  emotional eating, 192
  heart health, 184
  liver, 182–183
  for menopause condensed, 193
  phytoestrogens, 192–193
  simplified nutrition for wellness, 193–194
  systemic inflammation, 185

Organic Intelligence, 162
osteocalcin, 110. *See also* bones
osteocytes, 109. *See also* bones
osteogenesis, 109. *See also* bones
osteopenia, 109–110. *See also* bones
osteoporosis, 25, 110. *See also* bones
outside-in, 166–167
overwhelm, 168–169
oxygenation, 71–72
oxytocin, 20, 64

paced breath, 101. *See also* pranayama
Paleo-Yoga, 73
parasympathetic nervous system (PSNS), 130

passive stretching, 74. *See also* stretching
pelvic floor (PF), 142
  breath practices, 150
  changing biology, 142–143
  cobbler, 149
  core strength, 146–147, 151
  embodied connection, 151–153
  empowering pelvic health, 153
  exercises, 148–151
  genitourinary challenges in menopause, 143
  holding block, 148
  mula bandha, 144
  pelvic tuck, 148
  raised leg block hold, 149
  relaxing pelvic floor, 150
  teaching uddiyana bandha, 145–146
  uddiyana bandha or hypopressives, 145
  yoga for, 143–151
pelvic tuck, 148
perimenopause, 13, 14, 17, 21–24, 44–45
  emotional changes in, 163–164
  estrogen dominance, 23
  hormonal fluctuations, 23–24
  hormone therapy, 23
  mobility in, 55
  navigating trauma and emotional shifts, 51–53
  symptoms of, 22, 23
  systemic inflammation, 71
  unpredictable menopause graph, 22
  women safe spaces for, 44–45
PF. *See* pelvic floor
phytoestrogens, 192–193
pigeon pose, 82. *See also* stretching
pleasure and feel-good hormones, 63–64
PMDD. *See* pre-menstrual dysphoric disorder
PMS. *See* pre-menstrual syndrome
POI. *See* premature ovarian insufficiency; primary ovarian insufficiency

postmenopause, 13, 14, 17, 24–25, 45
posttraumatic stress (PTS), 65
posttraumatic stress disorder (PTSD), 65
postures. *See also* asanas/poses
    adjusting common, 112
    to avoid, 115
    and balance, 127
    reimagining yoga postures, 73–74
    restorative, 89, 106
    sloth posture, 62
    upside-down leopard on branch posture, 62
    from Yin yoga, 89
pranayama, 100. *See also* meditation
    boxed breath, 101
    breathing from research-based perspective, 101
    hot flashes, 100
    paced breath, 101
    seasons breath, 102
    sitali and sitkari pranayama, 101
    ujjayi pranayama, 101
    watercolour breath, 101–102
premature ovarian insufficiency (POI), 24, 195
pre-menstrual dysphoric disorder (PMDD), 21
pre-menstrual syndrome (PMS), 21
primary ovarian insufficiency (POI), 24, 195
progesterone, 19, 168
PSNS. *See* parasympathetic nervous system
PTS. *See* posttraumatic stress
PTSD. *See* posttraumatic stress disorder
pull-ups, 122

raised leg block hold, 149
reclining cobbler, 90–91. *See also* restorative yoga
relaxing pelvic floor, 150
reproductive aging, 17
reproductive hormones, 17
resistance bands, 119, 124
    band work for core, 126
    downward dog, 125
    locust pose, 125
    warrior I, 124
rest and vitality, 170–171
restorative yoga, 89. *See also* yoga class structure
    child's pose, 92
    favourite restoratives, 93–96
    inversion options, 94
    meridians, 96
    reclining cobbler, 90–91
    shavasana, 97–98
    Thai foot massage, 97–98
    twisted deer, 95
    Yin yoga, 89
    Yoga Nidra, 96–97
root lock, 81

sacroiliac joint (SIJ), 70
safer twisting, 114
sarcopenia, 72, 110. *See also* bones
seasons breath, 102. *See also* pranayama
seated positions, 99. *See also* meditation
self-advocacy meditation, 103–104. *See also* meditation
self-led movement, 69. *See also* mobility in perimenopause
serotonin, 20, 64
SFE. *See* spinal flexion exercises
shavasana, 97–98. *See also* restorative yoga
shifting mood, 165–166
side-angle pose, 87. *See also* stretching
SIJ. *See* sacroiliac joint
"silent disease". *See* osteoporosis
simplified nutrition for wellness, 193–194
sleep, 156
    causes of disruption, 156, 157
    CBT for, 161
    creating optimal environment, 157–158
sloth posture, 62. *See also* somatic movement
slow twist/washrag, 57. *See also* somatic movement
SMASHT, 182
SNS. *See* sympathetic nervous system

soluble fibers, 180
somatic, 55
somatic movement, 55. *See also* mobility in perimenopause
    angel twists, 58–59
    arm float, 56
    banana pose, 63
    sloth posture, 62
    slow twist/washrag, 57
    yes/no, 60–61
spaces meditation, 102–103. *See also* meditation
spinal flexion exercises (SFE), 112
spiritual fitness, 129. *See also* brain
stress, 27–29
    effects of chronic stress, 28
    posttraumatic stress, 65
stretching, 74
    adding muscular challenge, 86
    balancing poses, 83
    crescent lunge, 81
    dancer's pose, 84
    impact of forced stretching, 75
    half moon, 85
    hypermobility in perimenopause, 75
    intense side-stretch pose, 88
    muscular contraction types, 76
    muscular engagement in yoga practice, 76
    muscular inhibition, 74–75
    passive stretching, 74
    pigeon pose, 82
    side-angle pose, 87
    impact of stretching intensity on range of motion, 75
    triangle, 77–78
    warrior II and III, 79–80
sympathetic nervous system (SNS), 130
systemic inflammation, 71, 185
    free-radicals, 185–186
    nutrition, 185
    yoga for, 185

TA. *See* transversus abdominis
TCM. *See* traditional Chinese medicine

teaching language, 46, 48. *See also* yoga class structure
    challenging societal norms, 46
    menopause-sensitive yoga, 48–50
    spectrum of menopausal journeys, 47
    "The Change", 46
    trauma perspective on language and teaching, 50–54
tensegrity model, 41
testosterone, 20
Thai foot massage, 97–98. *See also* restorative yoga
"The Change", 46
thyroid health, 26
traditional Chinese medicine (TCM), 94, 96
transversus abdominis (TA), 146, 147
trauma, 50
    big-T Trauma, 51
    little-t trauma, 51
    perimenopause, 51–53
    -sensitive yoga teaching, 53–54
triangle, 77–78, 114. *See also* stretching
triceps curls, 122
twisted deer, 95. *See also* restorative yoga

uddiyana bandha, 145
    teaching, 145–146
upside-down leopard on branch posture, 62. *See also* somatic movement
urinary tract infections (UTIs), 142
UTIs. *See* urinary tract infections

vaginal "atrophy", 143
vagus nerve (VN), 130. *See also* brain
    vagal tone, 131
    yoga for, 131–132
vasomotor symptoms, 34
VCF. *See* vertebral compression fracture

vertebral compression fracture (VCF), 110, 112
vestibular-ocular reflex (VOR), 139
vestibular system challenges, 137–138. *See also* brain
VN. *See* vagus nerve
VOR. *See* vestibular-ocular reflex

warrior I, 124. *See also* resistance bands
warrior II, 79–80. *See also* stretching
warrior III, 79–80. *See also* stretching
washrag, 57. *See also* somatic movement
watercolour breath, 101–102. *See also* pranayama
weight-bearing exercise, 119
weight drills, 122
    lateral arm raises, 123
    pull-ups, 122
    triceps curls, 122
weight gain, 172–174
weights, 119, 120–121

yawn-stretch, 67. *See also* instinctual movement
yes/no, 60–61. *See also* somatic movement
Yin yoga, 89. *See also* restorative yoga
yoga, 31. *See also* restorative yoga
    challenges of research, 36
    dubious claims about, 34–35
    evidence-based reimagining, 35
    evidence for, 31–38
    health stereotypes, 39
    honoring feelings in, 164–165
    impact on menopause symptoms, 33
    intersection of yoga and menopause, 31–32
    before menopause, 32
    for menopause, 38–41
    menopause-friendly, 200–201
    menopause support, 32–33, 34, 35
    movement modality, 39
    for perimenopausal and later life, 45
    principles, 38, 39–40
    researched benefits, 37–38
    teachers, 201–202
    Yin, 89
yoga and lifestyle support, 155
    blood sugar regulation, 188–189
    digestive health, 177–181
    heart health, 183–184
    integrative approaches to menopause, 155
    liver, 181–183
    lymphatic system, 186–188
    protecting health, 177
    systemic inflammation, 185–186
yoga class structure, 43
    change in asana practice, 70
    language and compassionate communication, 46–54
    meditation and breath, 99–108
    mobility in perimenopause, 55–69
    open dialogue, 43–45
    restorative yoga, 89–98
Yoga Nidra, 96–97, 151–152. *See also* restorative yoga
yoga postures, reimagining, 73–74
yoga safety measures, 112. *See also* bones
    adjusting common postures, 112
    cat/cow, 113
    child's pose, 113
    common postures to avoid, 115
    downward-facing dog, 114
    getting to and from floor, 115
    half-wheel, 115
    option for those who can squat, 117
    safer twisting, 114
    supine, 116
    triangle, 114

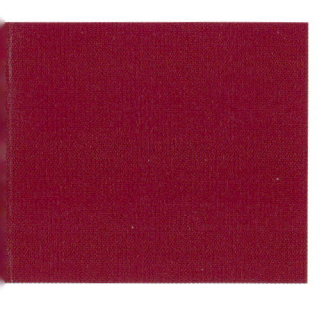

PEER REVIEWS

"This is a deeply personal and caring informative guide for both students peri- and postmenopausal, and for yoga teachers who work with them. Niamh Daly draws from her vast experience in dance, movement, Somatics, Alexander technique, Thai massage, nutrition, yoga and acting to offer a practical manual for yoga teachers. It includes important and relevant information on all stages of menopause as well as a realistic and a highly readable review of scientific evidence on yoga for menopause. This book offers teachers a comprehensive set of resource tools from pelvic floor health to emotional supports and from HRT to nutrition, and much more, to support and encourage students through the menopause journey. "Yoga for Menopause and Beyond, Guiding Teachers and Students Through Change" is a great toolbox on how to teach and perform specific postures with safety and functionality for everyday life as well as various pranayama techniques tailored to the needs of the menopause. It is a compassionate guide in self-acceptance for women, leading up to and through the menopause."

Dr Mary Flaherty, author of "Does Yoga Work? Answers from Science" and "Keys to Contentment from Science, Monks and My Mother"

"This is a really good reflective, interpretive view of the menopause transition with lots of practical calm guidance to help empower women."

Dr Annice Mukherjee

"Yoga is already recommended by all menopause societies as an evidence-based lifestyle intervention that can hugely help women. Here, Niamh has amped it up for menopause, and she is truly one of the best practitioners you can learn from. She continues to stay evidence-based, accurate, and diligent in her learnings and has a way of transferring her knowledge with kindness, humility, and grace to her students.

This book is going to be a game-changer for yoga practitioners throughout the world."

Amanda Thebe, fitness expert and author of "Menopocalypse"

"As a keen yoga student, Yoga for Menopause and Beyond is an enlightening read. It has given me choices and options for my practice, my life and wellbeing that are paving the way for me to be a proper bad-arse old woman, so I can age with more vitality, sass and discernment."

Kate Codrington, author of "Second Spring"

"Therapeutic insights to support the peri/menopausal phase have been missing from yoga curriculum for way too long and I'm so grateful that Niamh has created this valuable resource for yoga teachers! She has so eloquently blended traditional practices that have stood the test of time with a background in science & research, which is critical, in my opinion, alongside the clear gaps in information on perimenopause & menopause.

I'm so glad she has shifted our perspective with this supportive and empowering resource for all when most information on this topic is fraught with negative views & language on this precious wisdom bearing period of our lives.

Of course, this information is only helpful to us as yoga teachers & practitioners if it gets us to some useful therapeutic applications. These are well defined in this book, with plenty of detail on the applications of this information to our lives and our yoga practice. Thank you, Niamh!"

Tiffany Cruikshank, leading Yoga Teacher Trainer and founder of Yoga Medicine™

"Finally, a book that I can wholeheartedly recommend to women wanting to explore the ways that yoga can support, nourish, and smooth the oftentimes rocky transition into menopause and beyond. Although well meaning, so much of the yoga literature that has been published is steeped in misleading mythology; that certain postures can cure or ameliorate specific conditions, or that practicing deep forward bends, backbends, or unsupported inversions like headstand will address the myriad symptoms that arise at this time of life; hot flashes, disturbed sleep, anxiety, and fatigue. As Niamh Daly so bravely lays out, there's a paucity of evidence-based research to support these claims, and in some instances these practices can be injurious to women, especially those with osteopenia or osteoporosis.

In Yoga for Menopause and Beyond *you'll instead find clear and easy to understand explanations of the biochemistry of menopause and a sensible, accessible, and pleasurable approach to practice that will be inviting for women no matter what their level of experience. This is a book for real people in real bodies facing real challenges. Daly's immense experience in working compassionately with her students shows through on every page of this invaluable guide, from the delightful warm-ups that can entice an achy or fatigued body into movement; to the intelligent use of light weights in yoga postures, to the gentle supported restorative and breathing practices that can assist relaxation.*

Without making false promises, Daly conveys the immense benefits that can come from a balanced yoga practice as well as adopting simple lifestyle changes and sound dietary practices that can build overall good health. It is this broad-spectrum approach that can help to regulate the nervous system and help the body to find its own balance."

Donna Farhi, author of "Yoga, Mind, Body & Spirit" and "Bringing Yoga to Life"